#6 IN THE SERIES OF
BOOKS YOU'LL
ACTUALLY READ

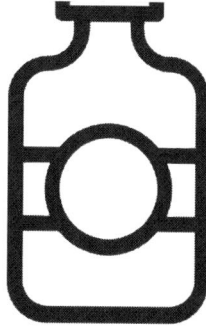

ESSENTIAL
OILS 101

DR. JIM BOB HAGGERTON

ANDREW EDWIN JENKINS

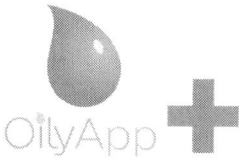

OilyApp **+**

A BOOK YOU'LL
ACTUALLY READ ABOUT
YOUNG LIVING'S
PREMIUM STARTER KIT!

ISBN number = 9781095054185 (black and white edition)

#6 in the series of books you'll actually read- go to www.OilyApp.com/books for more info about other titles.

Connect online!

Podcast-
OilyApp.com

Social-
www.Facebook.com/OilyApp
www.Instagram.com/OilyApp

Website-
OilyApp.com

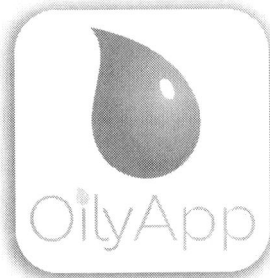

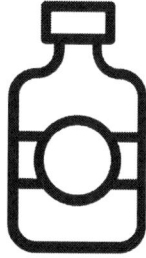

CONTENTS

AN OVERVIEW OF WHERE WE'RE HEADED!

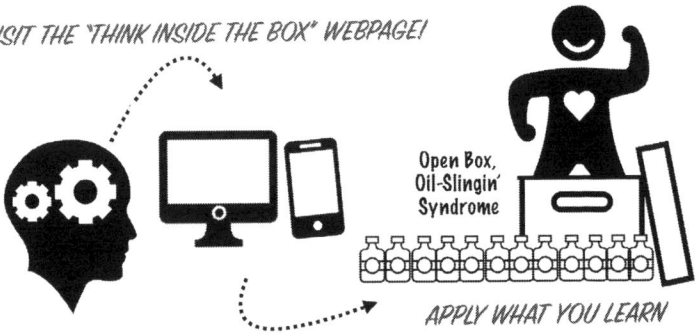

VISIT THE "THINK INSIDE THE BOX" WEBPAGE!

Open Box,
Oil-Slingin'
Syndrome

APPLY WHAT YOU LEARN

Exclusively at OilyApp.com/ThinkInsideTheBox

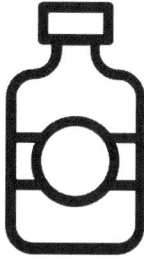

THE SHORT BOOKS SERIES AND ESSENTIAL OILS 101

Earlier this year we came up with an aggressive dream: *What if we cranked out one short book per month, something we could use to build our essential oil businesses, educate our team members, and help others understand the blessing of natural health we've stumbled into?*

The result was the OilyApp "books you'll actually read" series. That is, we decided to write short books that are scientifically solid, contain a lot of pictures, and make things radically simple. In other words, we intentionally place the "cookies on the bottom shelf," where people like us can read and understand everything.

We began by covering a few of the things we use every day- like the supplements (December 2018 release).

Then we dove into some topics we really love- like the Oils of Ancient Scripture collection, as well as the integration of supernatural healing and natural health (January 2019 release).

We wrote about life topics that hit us hard- things we learned *not* from reading books but from walking the tough terrain of the hard seasons of life. That took us straight to the Feelings Kit and the deep work of the soul (February 2019).

Then, we tackled that buzz word that floats around "home-based business world" like flies circling a summer picnic. Yes, I'm talking about *hustle*. People often assume you've got to make a calculated choice- that you can 1) set your family and personal life to the side and grind it for a season to succeed at work, or 2) you can set your business and financial goals to the side and succeed at home with your family. We discussed how you can do both, without losing your identity or attaching it to the wrong place (March 2019).

Finally, we took a hard look at Young Living's Thieves line. Shockingly, we discovered the company produces 25-plus Thieves products (April 2019).

That leads us to the topic of this book.

BACK TO THE BASICS

It's easy to forget where you began. For both of us, our journey into essential oils began with the Premium Starter Kit (PSK).

Yes, I ignored the natural health products in my house that others regularly used- with results- for over a decade (all while I gained 50 pounds and my health took a predictably quick nose dive). On a Young Living trip over 5 years ago, I caught a glimpse of my "festively plump" self in the mirror (that's the term I use) and thought, "Hmm… maybe I should give these products a try. Maybe I should actually try to be healthy by doing healthy things."

That led to a completely new chapter, a new outlook, and a new way of life. In fact, in the past five years *everything* has changed.

JB famously left his PSK sitting in a cabinet in the kitchen of his chiropractic clinic.

"Tucked away, it was just out of sight, out of mind" he said.

"You bought a kit and never used it?" I asked.

"A lot of people do. In fact, the stats say that over half of the people who order a kit won't ever order anything again. That means that many of us- as distributors- often don't do a great job of helping them understand what's in the kit. If they knew, they'd be using it."

"What made you finally pull your box of oils out and use them?"

JB was quick with the answer. "Our kids had a health need that none of our other tricks and tools were helping. Cindy told me to go get the box of oils."

"Did you remember where it was?"

"I actually had to think for a minute. But, yeah, eventually I found it. It had been there 6.5 years."

"What!? 6.5?!"

JB laughed. "Yeah. I was really busy. We were seeing 100 patients a day in our clinic. Life was just a grind."

"So what did you do, and what was the result?"

"Well," he continued, "I had to take the saran wrap off the box of oils. The diffuser had never even been used, so I had to figure out how to set it all up. But just twelve hours later, my kids were doing great."

"Hmmm… Young Living has this Seed to Seal promise," I said, "but you never unsealed the seal."

"Right. I suffered from Sealed Kit Syndrome."

THE CONDITION WE CLASSIFY AS SEALED KIT SYNDROME (SKS)

"I guess that's an actual thing," I told him. "I've heard stats like the ones you just mentioned. And I've seen people fall off my downline before. That means they stopped ordering, which means they weren't using the oils, which means that many of them probably never even got opened."

For JB, the oils did their thing. The rest- as they say- is history. You're reading his book and you've probably watched some of his videos online. But, you've only heard of him *now* because Cindy asked him to check that kit which he left sitting in the cabinet for almost 7 years. In other words, something caused him to overcome Sealed Kit Syndrome.

That's our goal for this book- to overcome Sealed Kit Syndrome (SKS). I'm capitalizing it, because it's a thing- a "legit condition" people fall into. *It's unintentional, but it happens, right?*

Now, let's *pause* right here. Let me explain who our audience is, so you know if this book is for you. We're writing to *three* audiences.

- First audience = We want to introduce you to essential oils in general and Young Living in particular.

- Second audience = You have a kit, and we want you to take the seal off it and begin using it. In other words, don't be like JB. Don't be like him in that respect, at least.

- Third audience = You've been around for a while, and you want to revisit the basics. You might have team members you're looking to train, or you want an easy on-ramp to lead others towards the lifestyle you've discovered.

I understand, you may be in group 1 and then move through group 2 fairly fast. Great. Either way, we want you to find yourself on the right side of that graphic! And, if you're in group 3, we want to help you move as many people as possible.

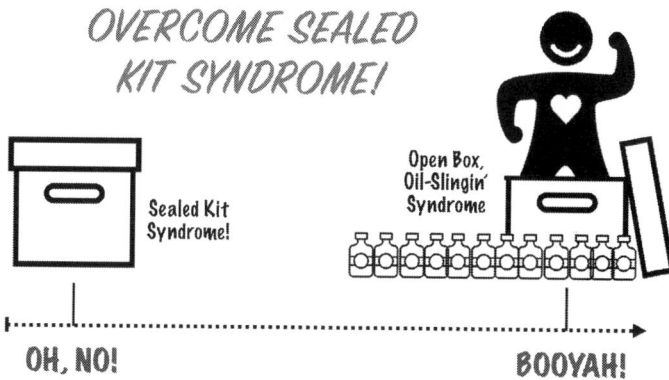

JB & ME, SOME HISTORICAL PERSPECTIVE

JB and I met at Advance 3.0 in Kansas City. We were both Platinum distributors at the time, which meant we'd been in the business long enough to have- let's call it what it is- some high level success. It's easy to get enamored with titles like Diamond, Crown, and Royal and forget that, at the end of the day, the average Platinum check is about $15,000 per month ($180,000 per year).

(No disrespect to the top tiers- I'm aiming all the way for the stars!)

Less than 0.1% of all people in the company hit Platinum. In fact, less than 0.1% of all people even attain the previous rank of Gold, meaning that if you're Platinum then you are, according to the Income Disclosure Statement, in the top 0.4% of all income earners via Young Living Essential Oils. At that level, you're earning more than most dentists, lawyers, and- candidly- most doctors. That's quite a feat.[1]

At that sweet place, though, it's easy to forget the basics. There's almost a natural tendency to try and make things more complex, to explore the "next level" products and dive deep into the compensation plan…

Success goes to your head (if you're not careful) and you get side-tracked. You lose sight of how things all began- that sacred spot where most people actually *still* begin.

BACK TO THE PSK

Fact: most people who join Young Living do so with the Premium Starter Kit (PSK). Yes, there are people who become members in others ways- and there always will be. Some will opt-in via Thieves, and others will join with Ningxia Red. Savvy and Slique kits opened more entry points. But the vast majority begin with the oils.

---

[1] Go to www.YoungLiving.com/IDS for the latest info on incomes, payouts, etc.

Not too long ago, JB and I discussed the PSK.

"I use it to teach *everything*" he said.

"What do you mean *everything*?"

"*Everything*. Everything is *everything*. I teach hormones with it. I teach digestion. I teach respiratory health and even other body systems. I teach people how to take care of things around the house- things like smelly laundry, funky odors from bathrooms and drafty places, spills and goo and other messes..."

I thought back to the past year. I'd taught classes on mental clarity, natural health, emotional health, and even men's health all by using the oils in the PSK alone.

"It's easy to forget how much that little box can do," I confessed.

"Yes, and most people start with that box. So, it makes sense that we start there and let them get comfortable with the oils and then begin exploring. Sure, we want them to add a few things that are unique to their situation, but we definitely need to show them the radical usability of that PSK."

NUTS & BOLTS, RADICAL USABILITY

So here we go. A book you'll read on the- we should trademark that term- *radical usability* of the PSK. All with the goal of breaking Sealed Kit Syndrome.

That said, let's get three housekeeping details out of the way.

First, it's easier to write in the first person. That is, it's easier to just *communicate* with you rather than trying to clarify who's talking, who said what, and in what order. So, since I'm the one sitting at the computer *today*, in this moment, you've got "first person Andy" for the rest of the book.

That said, you've *really* got me & JB. There's a lot of conversations, a stack of text messages, and a whole bunch of laughter tossed between these sentences.

As always, if it's science, *it's him*. Definitely him. If it's something else, it *might be* me. I'll try to recount the convos as closely as possible, so that you feel like you're sitting in the same room listening to the play-by-play with *both* of us. And, in many cases I'll recount specific conversations as closely as I can.

Second, let me offer you a few ways to use this book. Here are my top 3:

1. **Read it + review it + educate yourself on what's in the kit and add your own notes of other ways you can use it** (we've added notes space in chapter 4, during the run-down of each of the oils just for you!)

2. **Use the book to teach others about the oils.** Take it to the coffee shop, pass a handful of them around the room and let people follow along as you teach a class… we've printed this one in full color to make it- here's the term again- *radically usable*.

   At the end of the book we've included a few tips on how to lead your own class. You'll find it helpful to review that before using this book to lead others into their essential oil journey.

   Free tip: pass the books around the room before you begin teaching.

   Tell everyone, "Hey, I've got this great tool we're going to use. I won't read it to you, but I'll point to some pictures along the way, and show you places you might want to go back and learn more after you get your kit. At the end of our class, I'll take this back up. But, if you get your kit tonight, this will be a free gift for you to start your journey!"

3. **Send the book to your new members.** That is, keep a few on hand and physically send them a book in the mail.

   This book is a great tool for them to review. And, you can invite them to jump on the "Think Inside the Box" challenge we discuss in chapter 5.

   We've created a webpage specifically for that 21 Day Challenge, too, a quick journey that will lead people straight through everything in the kit.[2] They can read the info on the page- and watch a short video- or they can register to receive updates on their smartphone!

JOIN THE

21 DAY CHALLENGE

= THE BEST PREVENTION FOR SEALED KIT SYNDROME

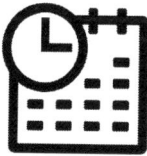

21 DAYS STRAIGHT + *3 THINGS EACH DAY* + *DELIVERED DAILY*

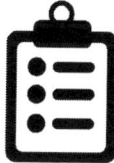

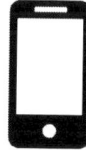

OilyApp.com/ThinkInsideTheBox

Third, I just mentioned it above- go to the website for this book. This book is a great tool, but so is the 21 Day Challenge.

---

[2] Go to OilyApp.com/ThinkInsideTheBox (the URL is case-sensitive, by the way).

- If you want an easy on-ramp to move from "zero to hero" in essential oil world…

- If you want great, practical tips you can share with others that will empower them to live their best life now…

- If you want step-by-step instructions on how to take those oils and that diffuser out of the box…

- If you want to join a community of like-minded people who are doing their best to move forward, together…

… then visit OilyApp.com/ThinkInsideTheBox and access the 21 Day Challenge.

Alright, let's get rockin'. Turn the page. JB and I have some great stuff for you!

All the best,

Andy

April 15, 2019

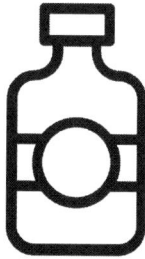

1 ESSENTIAL OILS DEFINED

MAIN IDEA= ESSENTIAL OILS ARE THE LIFE SOURCE OF THE PLANT. USUALLY DERIVED FROM STEAM DISTILLATION. MANY OILS HAVE THERAPEUTIC PROPERTIES THAT ASSIST YOUR BODY IN FUNCTIONING AT ITS OPTIMUM LEVEL.

You've probably heard of essential oils. You can order them online, you can buy them at the supermarket, you can even- get this- snag a few from Barnes & Noble or (gasp!) Walmart.

I'm not saying you *should* purchase them on clearance from a big box retailer. I'm just saying that it's *possible*. In fact, over the next few pages, I'll argue that you need to go for the absolute *highest* quality oil you can. After explaining *why*, I'll show you where to get them.

That said, you probably have *other* kinds of oils in your house right now- things like vegetable oil, peanut oil, and cooking oil. These oils are great for cooking and even eating. Some household oils can even keep lanterns burning when the power goes out.

Those types of oils are considered "fatty" oils. If you rub cooking oil on your body, it will clog your pores. It doesn't mean that it's a *bad* oil, it just means that is not its proper use- any more than the screen door was made for a submarine, as the old joke goes.

Essential oils are different than those oils…

WHAT THEY ARE = A SIMPLE DEFINITION OF ESSENTIAL OILS

Essential oils are volatile liquids which come from plants. They're often called *therapeutic* or *aromatic* oils. They're concentrated extracts from plants which help with some sort of function in our bodies.

Here's the non-scientific (read: *my*) version of what these essential / therapeutic / aromatic oils are:

> *Essential oils are the life source of the plant. Usually derived from steam distillation, many oils have therapeutic properties that assist your body in functioning at its optimum level.*

It's not thorough, but it helps me understand what they are, where they come from, and why different oils do different things.

Now, here's something that somebody smarter than me wrote:

> *Essential oils are volatile liquids and aromatic compounds found within the shrubs, flowers, trees, roots, bushes, and seeds that are usually extracted through steam distillation.*[3]

Here's a quick overview of what we just learned-

Essential oils are the life source of the plant = volatile substance derived from plants, containing the natural smell, characteristics and chemical compounds of the plant.

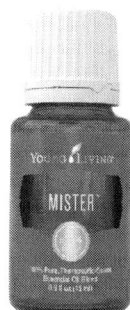

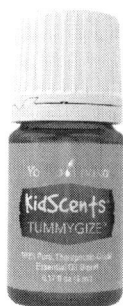

Essential oils are concentrated, and they're usually extracted through steam distillation, cold-pressing and resin tapping.

Essential oils are potent, volatile, & versatile. They have therapeutic qualities which can encourage, equip, and empower your health!

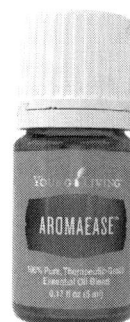

---

[3] *Essential Oils Pocket Reference*, p15. A similar quote appears on p1 of the reference guide, as well.

In chapter 4, we'll break down the Premium Starter Kit (PSK). I'll give you a list of twelve of the most popular oils and a brief overview of their best uses.

HOW THEY WORK = 3 CHARACTERISTICS OF ESSENTIAL OILS

Now that you know *what* they are, let's take a 30,000-foot fly-over and evaluate *how* the oils work. Consider this section of the book the equivalent of "Oils for Dummies."

The first thing you need to know about how essential oils work is that essential oils are *concentrated.* It takes a large volume of plant material to produce a small quantity of oil:

- 5,000 pounds of rose petals result in 1 kilo of rose oil.[4] A quick Google search revealed a kilo is about a liter.

- For every 2,000 pounds of grapefruit you distill, you'll net about 1.5 pounds of essential oil.[5]

- 2-3 tons of Melissa plant material produces just one pound of oil.[6]

In other words, it takes a lot of plant material to make a drop of oil, but a small drop of oil then contains the full force of the entire plant- *of all of those plants*.

---

[4] *Essential Oils Pocket Reference*, p1.

[5] "Core Vigor and Vitality" (in *School of Nature's Remedies* series), p3.

[6] *Essential Oils Desk Reference*, Fifth Edition, location 1.46.

When you have a bottle of rose oil, you have the life force of 5,000 pounds of roses. That's a lot of flower power. And that means a lot of life. Essential oils are *extremely* concentrated chemical compounds that pack a powerful punch.

CONCENTRATED

5,000 pounds ROSE *- 1 liter oil*

200 pounds GRAPEFRUIT *- 1 pound oil*

4,000- 6,000 pounds MELISSA *- 1 pound oil*

I asked JB if oils are like herbs.

"Kinda," he said. " I mean, they both come from plants. And they both have therapeutic properties. They're different, though. Way different."

I thought through what he said and then mentioned, "A lot of people have heard of- or are familiar with- herbs. They ask me all the time if essential oils are herbs. But I've never seen a liquid herb and I've never seen a dry essential oil."

"That's part of the difference. Herbs are generally dry, and oils are liquid" he replied. "But there are other differences, too."

While we talked, I grabbed my smartphone. Thanks to Apple's AirPods technology, I was able to talk to JB on the phone and surf the Internet at the same time. *Herbs*, according to Webster's, are "seed-producing plants that die at the end of their growing season and don't develop a persistent woody tissue. They disappear. Many of them can be used for "medicinal, savory, or aromatic qualities."[7]

In other words…

- Herbs are dead

- Herbs aren't concentrated

On the other hand,

- Essential oils aren't dead; they contain the life source of the plant

- Essential oils are concentrated

The result is that, "essential oils are 100 to 10,000 times more concentrated than herbs."[8]

JB clarified, "If people are getting results with herbs, they'll usually get far greater results with essential oils. They're more concentrated, so they're far more potent."

100 - 10,0000
TIMES   MORE   CONCENTRATED
THAN HERBS

---

[7] https://www.merriam-webster.com/dictionary/herb

[8] *Core Vigor and Vitality*, p3.

The second thing you need to know about how essential oils work is that their molecules are small. I'm not talking atomic particle small, but I'm talking small enough to slip and slide in and out of cells.

"They're kinda like little ninjas," JB said. "I know *ninja* isn't a scientific word at all, but they just get in and do their thing without you even seeing- or sometimes even feeling- them."

The *Essential Oil Pocket Reference* says that "Essential oils have a unique ability to penetrate cell membranes and diffuse throughout the blood and tissues…" They can do that, in large part, because they're tiny.

"So it's not just the liquid that you see?" I asked JB. "Rather, it's what's *inside* the oil you see?"

"Yes," he replied. "Remember, everything about them is concentrated."

Concentrated means that there's a lot of punch in a little package.

I looked at Dr. David Stewart's books, *The Chemistry of Essential Oils Made Simple* and *Healing Oils of the Bible*. Stewart suggests each drop of oil contains 40 million trillion molecules.[9] That's a 4 with 19 zeros after it. It looks like this:

40 MILLION TRILLION
MOLECULES   PER   DROP   OF   OIL

40,000,000,000,000,000,000

---

[9] *Healing Oils of the Bible*, pp27-28

By comparison, consider the composition of our bodies. Stewart reminds us that "we have 100 trillion cells... a lot."

When you look at how many molecules are in each drop- that's right, *a single drop* of essential oil, you get a better perspective. Stewart continues that "one drop of oil contains enough molecules to cover every cell in our body with 40,000 molecules."[10]

If you're a math person, here's your equation:

BASIC DIVISION- MOLECULES PER CELL

$$\text{Number of cells in body} \left] \dfrac{\overset{\textstyle\text{Molecules per cell}}{\text{Molecules per drop of oil}}}{} \right.$$

$$100{,}000{,}000{,}000{,}000 \left] \dfrac{\overset{\textstyle 40{,}000}{40{,}000{,}000{,}000{,}000{,}000{,}000}}{} \right.$$

Now, before making our third observation as to how they work, let's review what we've learned:

1. **Essential oils are concentrated.** It takes a *lot* of plant to produce just a *little* bit of oil, but that little bit has the life force of all of those plants combined.

---

10 David Stewart, *Healing Oils of the Bible*, pp27-28.

2. **Essential oil molecules are small.** And, there are a lot of them. They outnumber the molecules in your body enough to hit every cell 40,000 times with a single drop of oil.

That leads us to our third observation.

The third thing to know about how oils work is that they travel. Yes, they *move*. Let me give it to you in official language and then I'll give you an illustration. Gary Young, the founder of our company, wrote:

> When applied to the body by rubbing on the feet, essential oils will travel throughout the body and affect every cell, including the hair, within 20 minutes.[11]

All the way to your hair? From your feet?

Read the quote again. That's exactly what he penned.

Now, I know a guy whose wife swears that he used to snore. She rubbed Valor on the bottom of his feet one night, and the snoring- according to her- stopped that evening.

(He can't verify or deny it, because he always slept through his own log-sawing- same as most snorers.)

Pretty amazing, huh?

To sum up, the following three properties help us understand *how* essential oils work. They are-

- *Concentrated* (meaning "strong")

---

[11] *Aromatherapy*, Gary Young, p21.

- *Small* (meaning, they can go into tiny places)

- *Travelers* (put it anywhere on or in your body and it effects all of you)

ESSENTIAL OILS AREN'T NEW- A LOOK BACK AT HISTORY

All that said, essential oils aren't "new technology." They've seen a huge rise in popularity over the past five years, but they've been around for over 5,000![12] The therapeutic properties of plants have been used throughout history.

Most advanced civilizations have been using them since Creation. They are not an isolated phenomena. Researcher Scott Johnson writes,

> *Ancient texts and historical and archaeological evidence- including Egyptian hieroglyphics, Chinese manuscripts, Greek physicians' records, and Biblical references- suggest that essential oils have been an integral part of health and wellness for centuries.[13]*

Hippocrates is known as the "father of modern medicine." As part of their licensing process, medical doctors take the "Hippocratic Oath" as a promise to help and heal

---

12 I'm counting back, using the Hebrew calendar, as the Creation Story in the Hebrew Scriptures (also referred to by Christians as the Old Testament), is my starting point. The year 2019-2020 is year 5780. See https://www.science.co.il/israel/holidays/?y=5780 for more info.

13 Scott Johnson, *Surviving When Modern Medicine Fails*, p8.

the people they serve.[14] Notably, this famous Greek physician actually used essential oils as his medicines.

He wasn't the first, though. He was born around 500 BC. Ample evidence proves the Egyptians who lived a full thousand years before him integrated the oils into their daily routines. In 1819, a 900-foot long papyrus was found in Egypt, dating to 1500 BC. It is believed to be a "medicinal scroll," and contains over 800 herbal prescriptions and remedies as well as references to essential oils.[15]

In 1922, King Tut's tomb was discovered. The crew which explored the tomb found 50 alabaster jars (which would have held 7 liters of oil each, for a total of 350 liters total). Raiders had taken the oil but left the gold behind. Gary Young observed-

> The fact the gold reserves were left behind attests to the value of the precious oils that were once inside.[16]

He also suggested that "Kings would barter and buy land, gold, and slaves with their crudely extracted oils, because they were more valuable than gold."[17]

BRIEF BIBLE SHOUT OUT

Proverbs 21:20 tells us that "*There is* treasure to be desired and oil in the dwelling of the wise" (KJV).

---

[14] https://en.wikipedia.org/wiki/Hippocratic_Oath

[15] Gary Young, *An Introduction to Young Living Essential Oils*, p3

[16] Gary Young, *An Introduction to Young Living Essential Oils*, p3.

[17] Gary Young, *An Introduction to Young Living Essential Oils*, p3.

Let me give you some background on the verse. Solomon, the author of Proverbs, was the richest, wisest man to ever live. His wealth makes the Saudi sheiks, Warren Buffett, and Bill Gates look like upper middle class wage earners in comparison. Some economists estimate that if Solomon's wealth was calculated into current dollars, he would be a *trillionaire*- exponentially more than anybody on earth. In fact, you could probably add the top two guys together and Solomon would still surpass them combined.[18]

Tradition, as well as the Bible, says people traveled from all over the world just to listen to him talk (kinda like when JB hops online and goes "live"). And when they did, they stood amazed at his wisdom. Even with the little things like how his servants entered and exited the palace and how he conducted basic, everyday affairs, the guests were always impressed. They were spellbound, captivated by his knowledge and attention to every detail.[19]

The way he led his kingdom left them speechless, *because it all made so much sense.*[20] And, recall, this man just told us that oils are found in the homes of wise people.

(Solomon lived around 930 BC, by the way- about 500 years after the Egyptians and 500 years before Hippocrates.)

That said, we find over 200 references to essential oils in the Old Testament alone. And we see numerous references throughout the New Testament where Jesus instructed his disciples to anoint people with oil.

---

18 http://www.forbes.com/billionaires/ accessed 03-24-2014.

19 His story is found in 1 Kings 1-11.

20 1 Kings 10:1-13 details how this happened to the Queen of Sheba.

One of the first references we see is in the Creation story, though. Most modern translations tells us that God gave Adam and Eve every seed-bearing plant for food (Genesis 1:29). The word translated as "food" is the Hebrew work *oklah*, a word commonly used to refer to both "foods" and "medicines."

Though there was no sickness in the Garden of Eden, the inference is that God designed us to walk in health. And, He provided us with the resources in nature to do so. In other words, health isn't a "curse of the Fall" issue, it's our original design.

The Bible tells us that God is restoring all things- including the created order. In a vision, the prophet Ezekiel foresaw Heaven and a restored Eden. Using the same word *oklah*, notice he described the leaves (Ezekiel 47:12 NKJV, emphasis added):

> *Along the bank of the river, on this side and that, will grow all kinds of trees used for food; their leaves will not wither, and their fruit will not fail. They will bear fruit every month, because their water flows from the sanctuary. **Their fruit will be for food, and their leaves for medicine.***

Now, in Heaven no one is sick (Revelation 21:4). Everyone is well. However, like Eden, it seems that even there we're designed to walk in health.

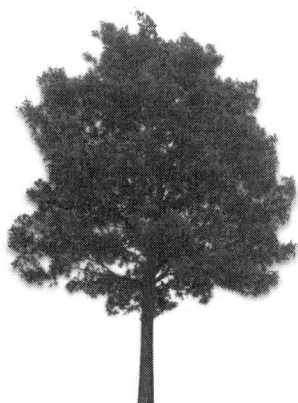

"THE LEAVES OF THE TREE... ARE FOR THERAPEUO..."
- *REVELATION 22:2*

Like Ezekiel, the Apostle John also saw into the future. Whereas Ezekiel communicated in Hebrew, John wrote in Greek. He also said, "the leaves of the tree are for the healing of the nations" (Revelation 22:2). Yet, due to the language differences, he wrote a different word.

You'll likely recognize the word he uses, *therapeuo*. Notice it in the graphic.

We have a similar word, *therapy*, which we use regularly. Sometimes we use the word to denote that we're overcoming a health challenge. Other times we use it to suggest we're proactively curbing something that could be an issue. Either way, though, the inference is that we're choosing to walk towards wholeness- in multiple areas of life.

Are there essential oils in Heaven?

I don't know. But I do know that they're derived from plants. And plants were given to us- according to the words of our Creator- to empower us to walk in our destiny.

In the next chapter we'll outline 3 ways you can use essential oils and we'll offer you a few safety tips- especially for pets and little people.

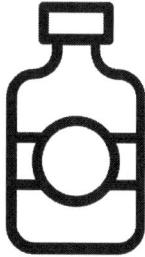

2 HOW TO USE ESSENTIAL OILS

MAIN IDEA= YOU CAN USE ESSENTIAL OILS TOPICALLY (TOUCH THEM) AROMATICALLY (SMELL THEM) OR INTERNALLY (INGEST/TASTE THEM).

Earlier in the book we talked about Sealed Kit Syndrome (SKS). I spent some time thinking about why people suffer from it.

Since JB was "patient #1" on this issue, I decided to just ask him point blank: "Why in the world would you spend hard-earned money on a kit and then just toss it in the back of a kitchen cabinet at your office, leaving it untouched *for years*."

He replied quickly. "Laziness and being too busy. We literally stuck it back there, and then I totally forgot we had it."

"I guess that's what happens to *a lot* when people get their kit," I said. "Their PSK usually arrives in the mail about 3-5 days after the class where they hear about it.

They receive a lot of new info during that first class they attend, and they forget it. Then they get busy…"

"Yeah," JB replied. "It's easy to just decide you'll open the kit and mess with it later. Most people haven't plugged in a diffuser before. They have a handful of oils that require a bit of brain power to sort through. There are a few things to figure out."

"I guess it's easy to punt it until after you get home from work. But then you come home tired and push it off a day or two…"

"And that day or two becomes 6.5 years," he admitted.

"I suppose," I continued, "that it would be completely different if essential oils were something people already use every day. It's almost like people are either nervous or afraid of diving into something new?"

"Maybe. You can go back to basics that people use every day. Pens and pencils don't come with instruction manuals," JB said. "People don't have to spend time and energy figuring out how to use them."

"But couldn't people just figure out the oils? I mean, people figure out complex things all the time," I replied. "Most Apple products don't come with instructions either. My kids learned to use an iPhone when they were 2. No manual needed."

"But you probably had to show your boys how to use toilet paper, right?"

"For sure. All parents know about those times when you go strip just-potty-trained toddler for bath time and you realize that, *oh, we've got to go do the wipe-after-you-go-lesson again*."

"Whatever the case, you learn to use pens because you see other people use them. You learn to use a smartphone because you watch other people do it. You don't necessarily learn to use toilet paper because you *don't* watch people use it. It's private. Essential oils kinda fall in that *you-don't-see-people-do-it-a-lot* category. You've got to, like a potty-trained toddler, be shown what to do."

Did you follow all of that? That's the caliber of convo you get when you have two guys steering the ship. You knew we would eventually get into poop and body functions, right?

That said, there are a lot of takeaways from that exchange.

- It takes a bit of time to "figure out" the oils- simply because they're not something we're used to working with every day. Nor do we "see" them as readily as we see other things we commonly use.

- The longer you put off opening that PSK, the easier it is to forget about the amazing goodness you have- all at your fingertips.

The purpose of this chapter is simple, then: show you *how* to use essential oils. We'll outline 3 ways you can apply them, and then we'll briefly discuss safety concerns.

1. TOUCH

The first of three ways you can use essential oils is super simple: rub them on your skin and let them do their thing.

Your skin is the largest organ in your body. And, it's full of holes, tiny pores which let sweat and toxins out and simultaneously allow other things in.

Remember what we learned in the previous chapter about oils being concentrated, small, traveling drops of goodness?

When they go *on* your skin, they move *into* your body. When they move into your body, they travel through your blood stream.

(This not only works for essential oils, this works for toxins in cleaning products and personal care products, too- which is why you want to make certain you use pure products everywhere in your home!)

Shortly after we received our kit in the mail, one of our boys slammed his bicycle into a telephone pole. I'm not sure if the front tire or his forehead hit the wooden beam first. Judging by the knot that began growing above his left eye, my guess is that he literally dove over the bars in order to save the bike.

We grabbed the Lavender, applied it directly to his skin, and let it do its thing.

That said, people often ask if essential oils are safe for kids.

I generally answer by telling them something like, "Essential oils are safer than Cheerios, over-the-counter vitamins with cartoons on them, and soda."

Once you understand how essential oils work- as well as how much sugar is in the cereal, the actual ingredients in over-the-counter "vitamins," and the immediate effects of soda, you "get it." Do the math. Some of the things we let our kids do are the health equivalents of playing in traffic.

When they look at me strange after receiving my answer, I just reply, "Yes, but it's best to dilute the oils for smaller people when you're applying them topically."

Here's how to dilute the oils:

- **First, find a high quality carrier oil**. Consider using Young Living's V-6 or opt for an organic coconut, avocado, olive, or jojoba oil.[21]

- **Second, dilute the oil based on the age of the child**. This decreases the intensity of the application.

Here are some helpful dilution ratios-

- **Birth to 6 months** = use 1 drop of oil + 1 tablespoon of carrier oil. Mix the two together in your hand and massage your baby.

- **6 months to 2 years old** = dilute the oil 4x the label's recommendation. For instance, if your toddler decides to play "chicken" with the coffee table and loses, take Lavender's recommended application of applying directly to the skin- but dilute it *times four*. That is, for every drop of Lavender you use, add 3 drops of carrier oil.

- **2 years to 5 years old** = dilute the oil with 3x the label's recommendation. That is, use 1 drop of oil per 2 drops of carrier.

- **5 years to 10 years old** = dilute the oils 2x. That is, use 1 drop of oil to 1 drop of carrier.

  Pro tip: Once you learn the oils each of your kids respond to most readily, go ahead and make a rollerball of a diluted mix.

  For instance, my 9-year old girl responds well to Eucalyptus Radiata. I ordered some empty bottles (and extra rollerballs). I keep a bottle in the drawer on her bedside table. It contains 30 drops of essential oil + 30 drops of Young Living's V6. This prevents me from having to mix

---

[21] V-6 = item number 3031 in your Virtual Office (VO).

something every time she needs it- and the rollerball makes spills non-existent!

Diluting the oils doesn't make them "less strong," anymore than wearing sunglasses makes solar rays less bright. Rather, the dilution filters the intensity, making the oil more palatable for small people.

Remember, skin is an organ- the largest one we have. You'll discover that everyone's skin is different, so everyone responds to the oils in their own way. It's often best to begin with a "less intense" version in the beginning.

DILUTION FOR KIDS

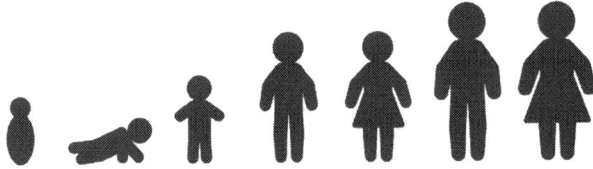

BIRTH - 6 MO	*6 MO - 2 YRS*	*2 - 5 YRS*	*5 - 10 YRS*
1 drop oil + Tbsp carrier oil	Dilute 4x label rec	Dilute 3x label rec	Dilute 2x label rec

Dilute w/ Young Living V-6, or Organic Coconut , Avocado, Virgin Olive, or Jojoba Oil

The same thing that's true for kids is also true for pets: they prefer a less intense version of the oils. If you're a "pet person," you'll notice that pets are incredibly sensitive to essential oils, responding quite nicely to them.

Many of the same uses for humans also work well for animals. Pet owners often diffuse oils like Valor for their furry friends during thunderstorms, and they regularly massage them with oils like Peace & Calming before visiting the vet (which is, in reality, a medical appointment!).

Instead of diluting the oils for your pets based on age, though, dilute their oils based on the size of your animal.

Regardless of the animal you want to serve, there are three size categories for dilution:

- **0 - 50 pounds** = 75% dilution = 1 drop of oil + 3 drops carrier

- **50 - 100 pounds** = 50% dilution = 1 drop + 1 drop

- **100 - 150 pounds** = 25% = 3 drops of oil + 1 drop carrier

You can use the same oils for dilution with pets that you use for humans. In addition, Young Living produces Animal Scents Ointment, which is part of their overall animal products collection.[22]

DILUTION FOR PETS

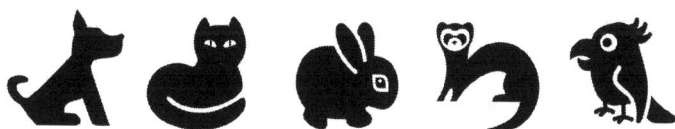

0-50 LBS = 75% dilution   **1 drop oil & 3 drops carrier**

50-100 LBS = 50% dilution   **1 drop oil & 1 drop carrier**

100-150 LBS = 25% dilution   **3 drops oil & 1 drop carrier**

Dilute w/
Young Living V-6
Organic Coconut Oil
Organic Virgin Olive Oil
Animal Scents Ointment

The dilution ratios are for topical application only. There's no need to dilute the oils when you're using them aromatically, that is, by inhaling them.

---

[22] Animal Scents Ointment = item number 5165.

2. SMELL

The second way you can use essential oils is to breathe them. Your skin is your largest organ, but your sense of smell is the strongest sense. It's tied to the limbic system, where memories and feelings are stored.

Your limbic system is why you can *smell* something- Fall leaves, apple pie, or even a specific perfume- and a memory instantly arises in your soul. It's also why hearing a certain song instantly transports you back to a different time and place. Your limbic system responds to words, smells, sound… all sensory input. Smell is the strongest, however.

Here's the scientific explanation:

> *When a fragrance is inhaled, the odor molecules travel up the nose where they are trapped by olfactory membranes… the lining of the nose…*
>
> *When stimulated by odor molecules, this lining of nerve cells triggers electrical impulses to the olfactory bulb in the brain.*[23]

The impulses are transmitted throughout the limbic system of the brain, throughout areas where taste, emotions, and even memories are handled. The limbic system is intertwined with the areas of the brain that control everything from your breathing to your heart rate to your stress load to your (or your wife's) libido! In other words, everything is connected.

---

[23] *Essential Oils Pocket Reference*, p25.

Again, smell is the strongest sense you have. And, since essential oils connect with your limbic brain when you breathe them, they carry the capacity to support your mood in the present, as well as heal emotional wounds from the past!

As we taught a class on the PSK one day, a friend of ours, a part-time nurse said, "I love to use Frankincense before starting my work weekend. It helps ground me and get me ready for a busy day."

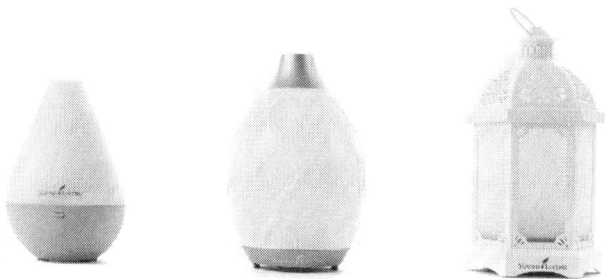

DIFFUSER + 4-5 DROPS OF OIL!

There are a few ways you can breathe the oils:

- Place 4-5 drops in a diffuser and let it run in the room while you're there

- Use a portable diffuser in your car or at your workstation

- Wear jewelry that acts as a diffuser (i.e., bracelet or necklace)

- Place a few drops in your palms, cup you hands, and breathe them

- Inhale directly from the bottle

Whatever method you choose- I recommend *all* of them- something special happens as your breathe.

What are some suggested uses for oils and breathing?

- Diffuse Lavender in your bedroom as you lay down to sleep

- Diffuse Frankincense as you sit to study or meditate & pray

- Diffuse Peace & Calming in a room where kids are acting a bit too rowdy

- Diffuse Peppermint and Lemon when you need a "pick me up."

- Diffuse Citrus Fresh to enhance the smell in certain "well used" rooms of your home

Do you see how this works?

This leads us to the third way you can use essential oils…

3. TASTE

Yes, the third way you can use essential oils is to ingest them. Now, two (brief, subtle, not intended to freak you out) words of caution before we discuss this third way to use the oils. I'll defy James Bond's wisdom to "never say never" on the first. And, I'll give you a definitive on the second.

- *Never* use a second-rate oil that you snagged from a bookstore, a big box retailer, or any place that specializes in anything except essential oils.

- *Always* use Vitality oils when you ingest. These oils are easy to spot as they're always dressed in white and trimmed with the same color as their "regular" oil counterparts.

A family friend named Rachel told me about her daughter's grumpy tummy. Seems like she couldn't get rid of the jitters, regardless of what she did.

"The school was calling me to get her every day," Rachel said. "And every day when I went to get her, she seemed so unhappy. I remembered the DiGize and Peppermint Vitality oils in the PSK, so I made her some capsules. I placed 3 drops of each oil in the capsules, diluting them with coconut oil. After trying for months to get her better with traditional methods- to no avail- in just a few short weeks with Young Living her tummy was supported back to its natural healthy digestion!"

What are the best ways to ingest the oils?

- *In a glass of water.* Place a few drops in a small glass of water and drink them. I do this with Citrus Fresh Vitality and Frankincense Vitality. Others use Lemon Vitality.

- *With a shot of Ningxia Red.* Place 2-3 drops in a shot glass of Ningxia Red (a full serving of Ningxia Red is 2 ounces). I do this every day with Thieves Vitality oil, as Thieves is my ongoing immune support.

- *In capsules.* Make your own capsules with oils you'd like to ingest- like Rachel did in the example above. For seasonal support, one of my daughters places 3 drops of Lavender Vitality, 3 drops of Lemon Vitality, and 3 drops of Peppermint Vitality in each capsule. She makes 10-15 capsules at a time, to insure she has enough for her week. [24]

- *In hot tea or coffee.* Place 2-3 drops of your favorite Vitality oil in your hot tea or coffee. Young Living carries everything from Cinnamon Bark to Lime to Orange (and even other flavors with which you can cook).

- *Drop directly into your mouth.* Place a few drops directly on your tongue- I do this with DiGize Vitality when I've had a bit too much kick in my food.

Here's an overview of the three ways we've covered-

THREE WAYS YOU CAN USE ESSENTIAL OILS

YOU CAN...	THIS MEANS THAT YOU...
TOUCH THEM	Apply them directly to your skin
BREATHE THEM	Smell them
SWALLOW THEM	Put them in a capsule, place a few drops in your mouth, or put a few drops in your favorite drink (tea or water)

BIG TIP: GET AS CLOSE AS POSSIBLE

Which way do you try first?

---

[24] Item 3193 = Clear Vegetable Capsules

Well, that depends on what you want to achieve. I use all three methods. I touch them, I breathe them, and I ingest them.

Here's what JB told me: "Get them as close to the part of your body you want to support. The oils travel, but go ahead and give them a head start."

He explained that if you're trying to enhance your mood, take advantage of the connection your limbic system and emotional center already has with your sense of smell. "Breathe the oils," he said. "Set up a diffuser wherever you are- in your home, in your car, in your office- and let it run."

"I've got a diffuser in just about every room in the house," I confessed.

"We do, too. And I usually have more than one of them going- because it's a great way to encourage yourself. Think about it…"

"And if it's something on your skin that you want to…"

"Just apply the oil directly to the part of your body that needs it. Again, get it as close to the place on you where you want it. Like the first rule of real estate: location, location, location."

"And if it's internal- like digestive support…"

"Then just make sure it's a Vitality oil and swallow it. Remember, though, you can ingest Vitality oils like Thieves for immune support. Anything that goes in your digestive system is pulled into your blood stream and circulates through your body. So think about ingesting other oils that benefit things happening inside your body, too."

As I continued putting all the pieces together, I told him, "It sounds like we want to use oils in all three ways, all the time, for sure."

"Yep. It's not a this or that or the other type of thing. Do it all. That's definitely the best way to go."

That said, now that you know the three ways you can use the oils, let's tackle one final topic in this chapter. Briefly, let's discuss essential oils and safety.

SAFETY = RED, YELLOW, OR GREEN LIGHT?

It always amazes me that many people think *nothing* about eating fast food (which is known to cause obesity and major health issues), taking pharmaceutical drugs (which contain laundry lists of possible side effects, including death), or using candles and cleaners (which admittedly are laced with chemicals). But, hand them an essential oil and they suddenly become hyper-health conscious and super-skeptical about everything!

"I need to do some research first," they say.

You've probably heard that line before. Shoot, you may have even (like me) said it!

Here's the sad irony, per "the research." According to the U.S. government, pharmaceutical drugs were one of the most common killers in 2018. Here's the death toll from four causes last year.

- 41,340 = drug overdoses from abuse

- 33,692 = traffic accidents

- 32,351 = guns

- 28,360 = falls

Those numbers are staggering.[25] What's more staggering, though, is that the number of deaths related to prescription use- not abuse, just *use*- topped 100,000.[26] At the same time, the number of reported deaths- or even serious illnesses- related to essential oils was *zero*. In other words, many people are looking at the wrong culprit in terms of how to make things safer. We look at political lightning rods- not necessarily reality.

That said, we've created an easy-to-remember way to determine which oils are safe to use and how to use them. Here are the three options:

- Red = stop, don't do it

- Yellow = pause, and proceed with caution if you decide to do it

- Green = full speed ahead

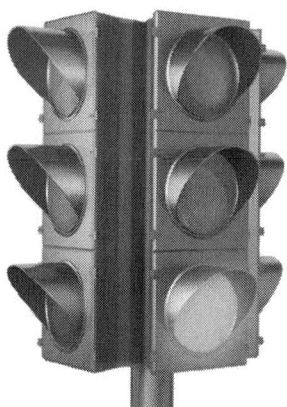

STOP!
1. Not in your eyes or ears
2. No styrofoam or plastic cups & straws
3. No mucus membranes

WAIT!
1. Pause before using on your face & sensitive skin
2. Look for safety caps & Vitality labels
3. Consider diluting if using on kids & pets

GO!
1. Instructions as written on the YL product label
2. 4-5 drops in your diffuser
3. White labels (Vitality) = internal, colored = external

---

[25] https://www.drugabuse.gov/related-topics/trends-statistics/infographics/drug-overdoses-kill-more-than-cars-guns-falling. See also https://www.washingtonexaminer.com/news/more-people-died-from-drug-overdoses-in-2017-than-guns-murders-or-car-accidents.

[26] https://healthfreedomidaho.org/prescription-drugs-kill-over-100000-people-each-year

Easy, right?

Now that you know how to use the oils- you just learned three ways to apply them- and you've got easy access to some safety tips- let's discuss what sets Young Living apart from all other companies. And, we'll define why that quality difference matters.

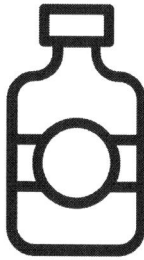

3 QUALITY MATTERS

MAIN IDEA= YOUNG LIVING CONTROLS THEIR PRODUCT FROM THE MOMENT THE SEED GOES INTO THE DIRT UNTIL THE GOODS ARRIVE IN YOUR HOME.

At one of the first Young Living events I ever attended, one of the company's global educators said something interesting.

"Everything that's labelled *'essential oil'* isn't the same," he said. "In fact, *it may or may not even be an essential oil at all.*"

Say what?!

I expected the YL exec to launch into a scientific explanation to further explain. However, Scott- the man who was speaking- explained that some companies aren't even trying to deceive you when they label their products as "pure." Sure, some clearly are. But, in his words, others "honestly have a different idea of what a pure oil is and what an adulterated oil is."

Purity is important, because if you purchase a product that isn't, you won't get the results you could get. Aside from the toxins and other chemicals you'll likely encounter by using an inferior product, impure oils just don't work.

RIGHT TOOL WORKS. WRONG ONE DOESN'T

Reminds me of something JB told me: "If you use something that's impure, you won't see the result you want. That might lead you to think that essential oils don't work. In reality, they do. You just happened to use something that didn't have the ability to achieve it."

"Kinda like trying to cut your front yard with a pair of scissors?"

"Yeah. It may do *something* beneficial- just like those sheers. You'll cut a few blades of grass. But as soon as you get to the other side of the yard, the stuff you cut first will be grown back. You'll never get ahead of it…"

"And the yard won't look even, it won't look right…"

"Yeah, you can draw that analogy out as far as you want. The problem is that inferior oils are the wrong tool for the job. We talked about the problems with toxins in our Thieves book. That's true whether you come in contact with toxin intentionally or unintentionally. Second rate oils have so many synthetics in them that I'm not even sure what they're the right job for."

I imagined myself walking into Home Depot, telling the yard guy that I needed something to trim my yard, and then being led to an aisle full of utility scissors. Rather than trying to mislead me or make a "dad joke," I envisioned the guy preaching the benefits of each brand of those scissors as we walked through the store.

A lot of companies are just like that hardware store salesman. They have no idea that those scissors- the second-rate oils- are the wrong tool. They understand that lawn mowers are better than scissors for cutting grass, but they don't understand that a higher quality oil is a better tool for anything related to your health and well-being.

If it sounds strange to you, think about it this way:

- Would you rather eat a burger from McDonalds or an Angus burger I cook for you on my grill?

- Would you rather drive a brand new Kia or a brand new Mercedes?

- Folgers or Starbucks?

- Coach or First Class?

See. We understand quality differentiation in every area of life. Essential oils are no different.

WHAT'S YOUR DEFINITION OF A "PURE" OIL?

At that YL event, Scott showed us a real life example- straight from company correspondence. A French exporter contacted Young Living about selling his oils. Because Young Living is the world industry leader in essential oils and has such a large market share, this type of thing happens quite regularly. Everyone wants a piece of that pie.

"The distiller proposed to sell Young Living 100% pure Lavender oil," Scott explained. "Then the gentleman defined what *pure* meant to him."

(Read this part carefully.)

The man's definition, straight from his email, read as follows: "(50% Lavender & 50% Lavandin) 100% pure."[27]

You don't have to know trig or calculus to understand that 50% of one thing and 50% of another is *not* 100% of one thing. It's *not* pure. It's cut. *By half.*

The man sending the proposal wasn't trying to deceive anyone- *he was totally honest about what he was selling*. But, his definition of *pure* is different than yours and mine. And that makes a huge difference when you're talking about what an essential oil can do.

In the first chapter we learned three things about essential oils: concentrated, small, travelers. If you add *anything* to them, you change the three factors which make them capable of doing their job! At the same time, you might actually add something back that makes the oil ineffective.

Here's what I mean…

Scott explained that Lavandin, the added ingredient the salesman was using for 50% of his "pure" oil, often causes skin irritation. Lavandin is a cross between Lavender and Spike Lavender, and it contains a compound known as Camphor.[28] Lavender is great for regulating circulation and the bleeding process along with supporting bumps and scrapes. It's definitely one to keep handy for when you

---

27 "Core Vigor and Vitality" (in *School of Nature's Remedies* series), p5. The email text is included on that page.

28 To use the terms we learned earlier in the book, the vendor was selling a blend- and not a single oil. He was not selling a synthetic.

have spent too much time in the sun! If you put Lavandin on your skin when it's sensitive, though, the camphor might cause inflammation.[29]

Scott said, "This might lead you to think- again- that essential oils simply *don't work*, when the issue wasn't the lavender at all- it was the extra ingredient."

Make sense?

He mentioned another scenario that plays out when potential suppliers call Young Living.

Young Living will often say something like, "Sure, send us a sample. We'll test it in our lab and get back to you."

The next question that often comes from the vendor is, "What do you want it to *smell* like?"

Scott offered the hypothetical response that YL kicks back, "What do you mean, *'What do we want it to smell like?'* We want it to smell like whatever the plant really smells like!"

Over the past 5 years I've smelled most of the oils. We received a $1,900 kit chock full of oils for hitting the "Silver in Six" rank as a distributor.[30] The day the oils arrived, we sat in the living room and smelled *all* of them.

Honestly, I love how some of them smell. Others, well, let's just say I didn't care for them as much. But I understand they *all* have therapeutic uses, meaning they each provide health benefits. And I know that *Young Living oils all smell like what they*

---

[29] Source: Scott Johnson, private message, 04-07-2014.

[30] This was a program Young Living used to have to encourage business building. The program has changed to an even better program whereby you can win some amazing prizes- all while working at a paced plan of business growth. We included a video of the Elite Express in the January 2019 edition of OilyApp+ - go to www.OilyApp.com and login.

should smell like. The oils smell like whatever the plant produces. They don't smell like a preferred scent that someone created in a lab and then injected into the oils, thereby diluting it, and making it more pleasant to the olfactory palette.

ALL OILS AREN'T EQUAL- 3 GRADES

This leads us to a major point about oils: **all essential oils are- obviously- *not* created equally**. The *Essential Oils Pocket Reference* contrasts two qualities of essential oils: *aromatherapy* grade and *therapeutic* grade.

Aromatherapy grade oils are cheaper than therapeutic grade oils. They are watered-down, the essential parts of them are stretched to fill more bottles, and they have added fillers (i.e., fragrances). You can't ingest them, and the label on the bottle will say so. In fact, when you're in doubt you can always read the instructions!

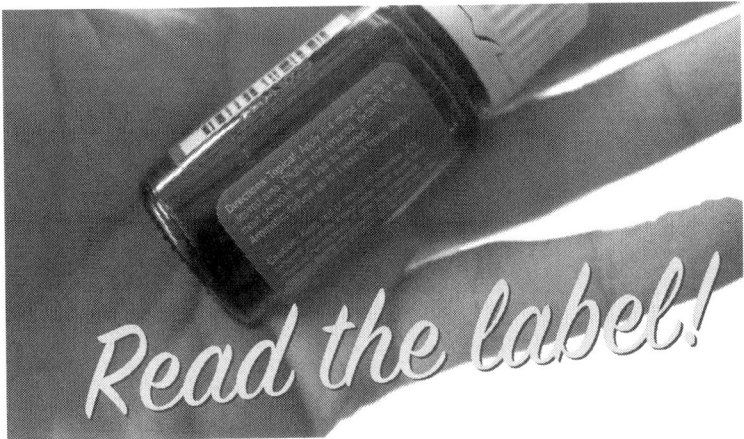

Read the label!

Because of all of the additives, aromatherapy grade oils have a weakened ability to travel. The impurities bonded to them make them larger than they should be. And, they're not as strong. In other words, none of the three properties we discussed in chapter 1- concentrated, small, travelers- are true of aromatherapy grade oils.

The name is tricky. The word *aromatherapy* actually sounds legit- like it's important, scientific, and powerful.

And, in other countries (like France, for example), you'll find certified *Aromatherapists* who are trained, credentialed, and able to help people with… get this… therapeutic grade products. In other words, the word *aromatherapy* often means something totally different over here than it does over there.

Therapeutic grade oils, on the other hand, are *pure*. There is *nothing* added to them at all. You only get the aromatic, volatile substance of the original plant. Therefore, you can actually ingest many therapeutic grade oils (i.e., as we discussed in chapter 2, you can place drops of it in a capsule and swallow it, you can drop it in water and drink it). You should *never* do that with a lower-grade oil, however.

(Pro tip: Not all therapeutic grade oils should be ingested. Young Living always recommends consulting with your primary medical care provider before ingesting therapeutic grade essential oils if you are pregnant, nursing or have other medical conditions. And, Young Living places white Vitality labels on oils fit for ingestion.)

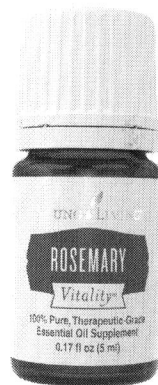

You need to research the oil producer and find out if, like the Frenchman in the Lavender example above, his definition of *pure* is the same as yours. Some manufacturers promote their oils as "pure" when they clearly aren't. Again, sometimes this is intentional deception, sometimes it's not.

I'm not judging their motivation for "cutting" the purity of the oil, I'm simply stating the raw fact. Most manufactures do it. To be clear, "Young Living offers pure and authentic oils *as close to how they are found in their natural and living state as possible.*"[31]

By contrast, Daniel Penoel, who writes the forward for Gary's book *An Introduction to Young Living Essential Oils*, says,

> *Many companies have jumped onto the aromatic bandwagon solely for commercial reasons. They simply do not know the meaning of genuine when it is applied to essential oils. They market products that are made solely for what I call recreational fragrancing.*[32]

Recreational fragrancing? Yes, *recreational.*

I told you about two categories above: *aromatherapy* grade and *therapeutic* grade. I would add a third category of oils: *novelty* grade.

There's a shop in 5 Points South near downtown Birmingham, a local intersection that has a few clubs, a coffee shop, several restaurants, and an undefined shop where you can purchase old records, hipster clothes, and drug paraphernalia- for "display purposes only," of course.

They sell incense sticks in that shop at the meager price of "5 for $1." Light them, and the smell rises with a tiny, winding smoke stream. You can buy Cinnamon sticks, Peppermint, Lemongrass, Patchouli, Juniper, and Fennel- among other types. They sell oils by the same name- for $5 a bottle or "5 for $20." Notice, they have the *same names* as the essential oils YL manufactures.

---

31 "Core Vigor and Vitality" (in *School of Nature's Remedies* series), p5.

32 Gary Young, *An Introduction to Young Living Essential Oils*, iii.

There is nothing "essential" about any of their oils and sticks, though. They *might* smell good, but they don't qualify as aromatherapeutic or therapeutic. They're *novelty. Recreational. Period.*

Here's a visual-

QUALITY CONTINUUM- 3 GRADES OF OILS

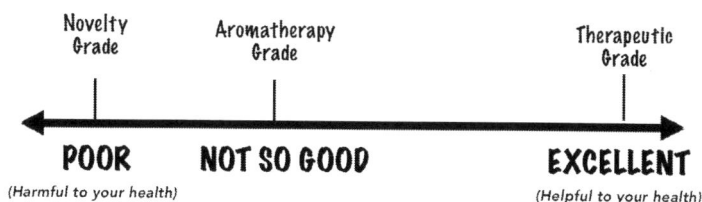

Novelty Grade	Aromatherapy Grade		Therapeutic Grade

$$\longleftrightarrow$$

POOR	**NOT SO GOOD**	**EXCELLENT**
(Harmful to your health)		(Helpful to your health)

Remember, a few pages ago I mentioned to you that the essential oils contain the "life force" of the original plant. I know, it sounds New Age or Star Wars-ish, but once you understand the truth of it, a lot of things start making complete sense. You start understanding why the oils work. And you start really seeing why you want pure oils instead of half-breeds (aromatherapy grade). Or even non-breeds (novelty grade).

Those are *not* essential oils, even though they may be marketed as such. As you become more and more familiar with pure essential oils and how they're sourced, you'll see that "a large percentage of essential oils marketed in the United States fall in this adulterated category."[33]

---

[33] *Essential Oils Desk Reference*, Fifth Edition, location 1.4.

CLARIFYING QUESTIONS- MAKE IT PRACTICAL

Before going further, let's answer three questions. Asking- and honestly-answering these will help us further see the importance of using a better product.

Question 1: Where do the oils sold at Barnes & Noble, Target, and Walmart fall on the spectrum?

Answer: While some oils you find in health food stores might be aromatherapy grade, the oils you find the majority of the time are recreational grade.

Think logically here:

- Barnes & Noble is in the book business- not natural health.

- Walmart doesn't sell "high-end" anything. They don't sell top tier athletic shoes, designer fashions, or the best personal care products. We buy things at Walmart because we can find *certain* things- but not all things- drastically cheaper.

Question 2: Why would someone alter the oils? Why doesn't everyone just make a better product.

Answer: First, some people don't know better. Again, go back to the example with which we began this chapter. The Frenchman wasn't trying to trick anyone. And Walmart might not be, either. Some sellers legitimately don't know the benefits of full strength oils.

Second, there are other, obvious reasons creators might alter their oils:

- The profit margin is higher if you stretch the product

- More consumers *will* buy a cheaper product when offered to them (assuming they don't understand the quality disparity, who wants to spend $25 on one bottle when they can buy *five* for $20?)

- The shelf life is longer (food people have known this for years- hence, all the additives and preservatives)

- You can control the final product, insuring it always smells the same and that you never run out of inventory.

Question 3: Will lesser grade oils help me?

Answer: You might receive *some* benefit from aromatherapy grade oils. We purchased oils off the shelves of health stores for years- and got some measurable results. However, we were blown away by the results we received with pure oils. There was no comparison. If you're benefiting in any way whatsoever from a lesser quality product, consider the exponential benefit of moving to a better grade.

Here's a final review of the 3 grades of oils we discussed.

COMPARISON OF THE 3 GRADES OF OILS

GRADE	CHARACTERISTIC	WHAT IT MEANS
RECREATIONAL GRADE OILS	Is basically a liquid with a synthetic smell added. These are for entertainment value- or symbolism- only.	They are actually harmful as they are toxic (which is why your body reacts to the smell, often).
AROMATHERAPY GRADE OILS	Have "fillers" that have been added to make them stretch and fill more bottles.	They simply do not work as well, so you may not actually get any benefit. This might lead you to think that "essential oils" don't work (when, really, you just used an inferior product).
THERAPEUTIC GRADE OILS	These are pure. If it doesn't grow, you don't get it.	Your body can make use of these, because they are natural and pure.

JB RANTS ABOUT QUALITY

Young Living has been the world leader in essential oils for over 25 years.

JB told me, "My wife and I are both licensed chiropractors. There's a reason why we've *exclusively* used and recommended Young Living oils and products above all other companies for more than a decade."

"Is it all of that science stuff we just discussed?" I asked.

"Sure. All of that is part of it. The integrity of the product, it being the highest of the three grades… It all comes down to this one word, though: *quality*."

"Somebody asked me about Young Living and why we didn't just go with another company…" I told him. "They inferred that other companies that referred to their oils as 'therapeutic grade' were the same."

"Those are all copy-cats," JB said. "They're all trying to mimic Young Living, because Young Living is the original and consistent forerunner in the industry."

"Well," I added, "I don't know if this is a good analogy or not, but I likened it to this for that person… My boys love Chik-fil-A. Every chance they get, they want to eat there. Chik-fil-A has this saying: 'We didn't invent the chicken, just the chicken sandwich.' I kinda think the same thing about Young Living."

"True. Gary didn't invent essential oils. They've been around for- literally- millennia. He studied for years in France, which was somewhat of the epicenter of oils for the last century. That's part of his legacy. However, he is the one who took oils into this next era of absolute purity and testing standards to insure that quality expectations are met. This is what enables the oils to work like they're supposed to."

"I've heard stories about Gary dumping entire batches of oil because they didn't test out right."

"That's true. There are times when the oil met industry standards but not Young Living's standards- which are even higher. So, he refused to take the product back to the market."

"When we first began using Young Living about five years ago, " I said, "one of my favorites was Valor. Still is. But that oil went out of stock for 2-3 years."

"Yeah, a lot of companies boast that they *never* run out of stock. When you're not worried about quality, you can say that. But when you have a naturally grown product that you can't get until it harvests, you have to wait for it to grow. And then you have to check and make sure the product meets quality control..."

JB continued, "Then there's this. It's one thing to make sure the oils you get for your company are *pure*. Most companies don't do that. It's an entirely other thing, though, to have the testing capability to ensure exact standards on the potency and therapeutic quality of all of the constituents within the oil."

"Explain why that matters," I said.

"Well, you can have a pure oil- that means the only thing in it is the oil. No fillers. No additives. No synthetics. But, if it wasn't grown at the right pH or harvested too early..."

"I've heard about this. I've heard different plants need to be picked at different times for maximum effectiveness, and that others need to be distilled in certain ways..."

"Yes. Otherwise, you may end up with an oil that looks and smells amazing... but it has absolutely no therapeutic affect when you use it."

"Is Young Living the only company that can ensure this quality?" I asked.

"They are. Before Gary died, one of his legacies is that he developed the largest library of essential oil samples for testing in the entire world."

"What does that mean?"

"Well, the company uses a GCMS- a Gas Chromatography Mass Spectrometer…"

"A what?"

"It's a fancy machine that tests an essential oil and then charts the components into a graph. You can see what's in the oil by percentage. This allows you to determine if the volatile ingredients- the things that make it work- are in there."

"Couldn't other companies just buy one of those?"

"If they could afford it, yes. But then what would they compare their tests to? Our library of oils gives us a plumb line to go back to."

"Gotcha. That make sense…"

"There's more, though. Young Living has two more GCMS-2 testers. Those are more in depth than the first machine. If it doesn't pass the first test, it's tossed. We don't ship it. But then we go through more testing."

"What do people need to take away from this?"

"A few things," JB said. Then, he began his rant- "First, a lot of companies use buzz words like *organic* and *pure*. Those words don't mean much unless you can actually test the final product."

"I've heard that something can be labelled *organic* if 95% of the ingredients are organic. In other words, it just has to be a majority of what's in there. It could be 5% totally harmful."

"That's true. And that's why you need to test everything to see what is actually in the product. And you need a process that you oversee which insures you'll hit that target. The test shouldn't be a 'let's-hope-this-makes-it type of thing. Rather, that test should confirm what you thought would be true, yet catch something when it's not."

"What do you mean?"

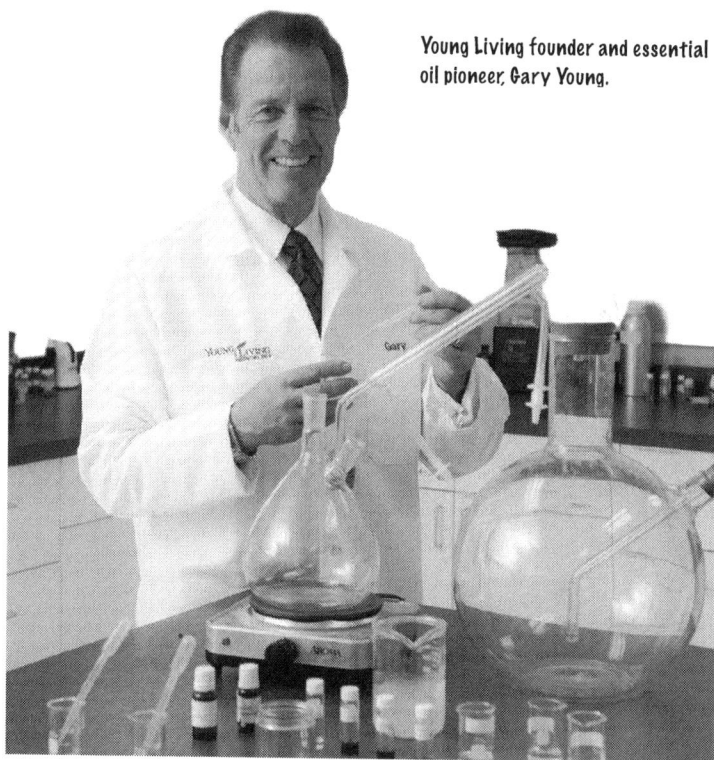

Young Living founder and essential oil pioneer, Gary Young.

"Well, Young Living has the Seed to Seal process. They've got the SeedToSeal.com website that explains it in detail. Seed to Seal is Young Living's process to begin with a Seed, Cultivate the plant, Harvest it in the right way, Test it in the lab, and then Seal it before sending it to you. Those are the five steps…"

"Seed, Cultivate, Harvest, Test, Seal?"

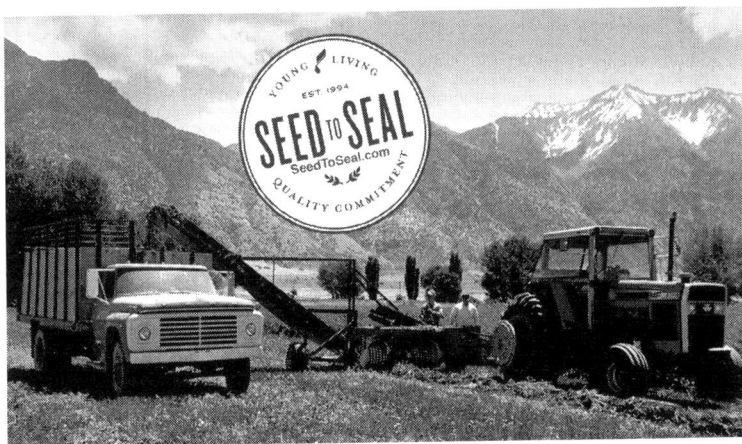

"Yes. Even if you forget the five words, the important thing to remember is that *Young Living is the only company that controls that entire process.* They're the only company that owns and operates their own farms- and works so closely with partner farms that you can go walk on the farms yourself, right now.[34] They have that much control over it and are that transparent. So, when Young Living runs a test, they're not merely *hoping* the oil will pass, they have a strong idea that it's going to. They've controlled the entire product for those first three steps…"

"But if it doesn't pass that fourth step, the Test…"

---

34 http://seedtoseal.com/en/global-farms

"Then they toss it," JB said. "They dump the oil."

"And we have something to compare it to because we have the oil library and all of the data that no one else has?"

"Right. No one tests like we do. Even if they did, they don't have the library to verify anything. And they don't oversee that entire process."

"What else do people need to know?" I asked.

"Well, Young Living does an incredible job of getting the product from the Seed to the Seal. That's their guarantee. They plant, cultivate, harvest, and test with that in mind. The process isn't about the test. It's about the final Seal- about getting the best possible product on the planet to you."

"So what's the next issue?"

"You've got to unseal what they seal in order to use it. Young Living goes Seed to Seal…"

"But then you've got to get past Sealed Kit Syndrome."

"Yes. The oils don't do anything for you sitting in a kitchen cabinet in the break room at the office."

"That's where we need to go next, then. We've told them what oils are, we've outlined how to use them in general, and we've outlined the quality issue- and why it matters. Next, we need to talk through the specific way to use specific oils…"

"Next chapter, let's do it."

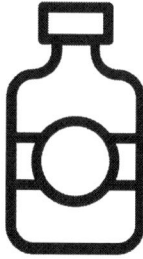

4 TWELVE OILS AND MORE

MAIN IDEA= THE EASIEST WAY TO BEGIN YOUR ESSENTIAL OIL JOURNEY IS WITH YOUNG LIVING'S PREMIUM STARTER KIT. A DIFFUSER, 12 OF THE MOST POPULAR OILS, AND A COMBO OF BONUS ITEMS CREATE THE PERFECT JUMP-START!

I asked JB the best way to start a journey with essential oils: "So let's say somebody wants to begin their journey. They're sold on what oils are- like we hit in chapter 1. They understand the three ways to use them- like we talked about in chapter 2. And they realize they'll get a real result with a therapeutic grade oil- like we just explained in chapter 3. *How do they know what to order? How do they know where to begin?"*

"If they want essential oils, they should order Young Living's Premium Starter Kit. It has everything they need to begin. And it's a great launching pad to help them go further."

We walked through the PSK- Premium Starter Kit- for about an hour.

JB reminded me, "The PSK comes with 12 oils and a diffuser. The diffuser, valued at about $80 means they can use all of the oils in that kit the second way we discussed, by inhaling them. In other words, they can create a calmer, more relaxing atmosphere the moment they receive the kit."

"It used to come with just 11 oils, back when I first began using the products," I said.

"Me, too. But they added an additional oil for 2019."

As we spoke, I made a few notes in my sketchpad. Below, I've provided you with a cleaner version of the chart I drew (you wouldn't be able to read my writing, trust me). The chart will make more sense after we work through this chapter.

OVERVIEW OF PSK OILS

OIL	SINGLE (4)	BLEND (8)	VITALITY (5)	REGULAR (7)	SAFETY CAP (1)
CITRUS FRESH		YES	YES		
DIGIZE		YES	YES		
FRANKINCENSE	YES			YES	
LAVENDER	YES			YES	
LEMON	YES		YES		
PANAWAY		YES		YES	YES
PEACE & CALMING		YES		YES	
PEPPERMINT	YES		YES		
RAVEN		YES		YES	
STRESS AWAY		YES		YES	
THIEVES		YES	YES		
VALOR		YES		YES	

Look at the chart to your left.

The PSK includes 4 singles and 8 blends (first two columns). A single comes from one plant, and a blend comes from multiple plants. Since so many oils work so well together, for convenience Young Living bottles many of these for us. A bottle contains a single or a blend- but not both.

Of those 12 oils, 5 are Vitality oils (labeled for ingestion), 7 are regular oils. An oil is either a Vitality oil or it's not. (Remember, Young Living produces some of the same oils- like Frankincense- in both a Vitality and a "regular" version.)

The PSK also comes with 2 servings of Young Living's propriety Ningxia Red, as well as enough concentrated Thieves Household Cleaner to make a full bottle.

Over the next 20-plus pages, we'll walk through the oils. You'll see pictures and bullet points, making it incredibly easy to see how to use each product.

I'll provide you with space to jot your own ideas and make notes. As you read, though, I'd like to ask you to do so with an open mind, looking for specific areas in your life you'd like to see something change for the better.

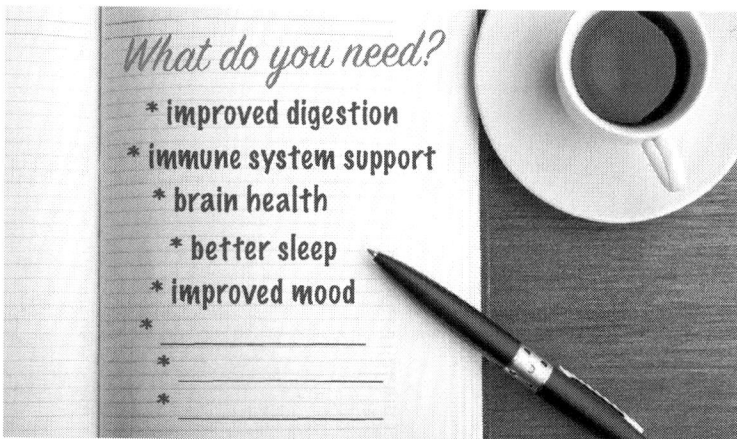

What do you need?
* improved digestion
* immune system support
* brain health
* better sleep
* improved mood
* _____
* _____
* _____

CITRUS FRESH

Happy smelling home!

Great with laundry

Shoes, closets, cabinets

Mood booster!

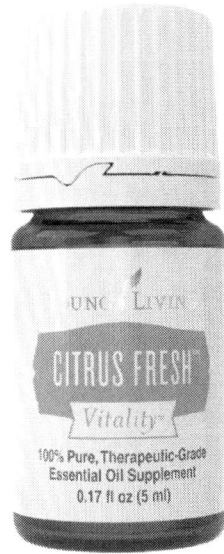

Single or blend: Blend, containing all the goodness of 6 citrus plants

Vitality: Yes

Suggested uses:

- Diffuse for an uplifting scent

- For stinky shoes, place 2-3 drops on a cotton ball and roll to the middle of the shoe

- Great for gym clothes or soured laundry- add 2-3 drops to your detergent in order to curb the undesirable smell

- Add a few drops to your cleaning agent

- Add 2-3drops to your lotion or moisturizer to boost your skin care routine

Odd fact, tidbit, random info: Fragrances from candles, scented air fresheners, and even household cleaning products are known to contain carcinogens. Increasingly, people are viewing them to be as dangerous as secondhand smoke. Do a quick Google search to learn more about how Citrus Fresh provides you with one of the many healthy Young Living alternatives.

NOTES

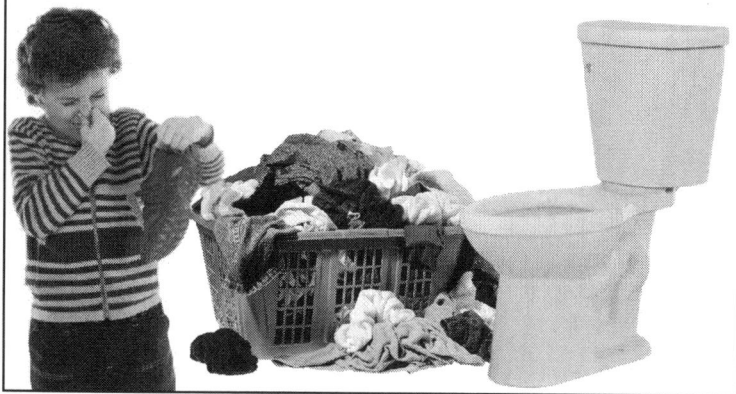

DIGIZE

Gold-standard tummy support

Traveling intestines

Two words: spicy food

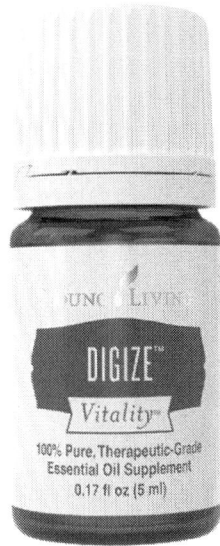

Single or blend: Blend

Vitality: Yes

Suggested uses: DiGize is the gold standard in immune support.

- Place 2-3 drops in a glass of water and drink before you eat "challenging" food (to help with bloating and digestion)

- Place 2-3 drops on your tongue while in a restaurant, after eating or make your own capsules to have on hand

- Rub directly on your belly

- Diffuse if needed

Odd fact, tidbit, random info: The smell of Digize is… well… unique. However, in time the characteristic smell will remind you of- and signify to your body- that digestive support is on the way.

NOTES

Pro tip: Use the names of the oils with your kids and tell them how you are using them. After working his way through that stack, Salter asked for DiGize by name!

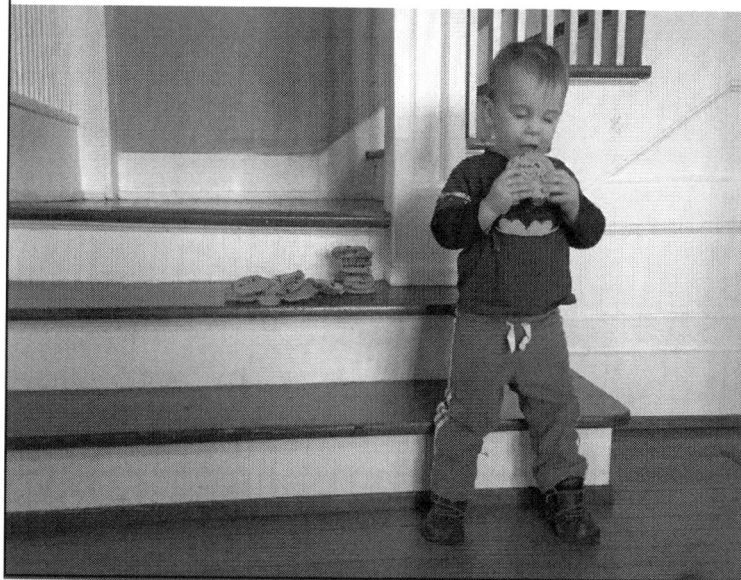

FRANKINCENSE

Mood lifting

Inspiring

Awesome skin oil

Focus & concentration

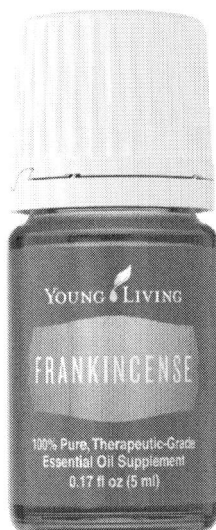

Single or blend: Single

Vitality: No- but Young Living produces Frankincense Vitality

Suggested uses: Ancient Egyptians said, "Frankincense is good for everything from head to toe."

- Brain focus & clarity = diffuse or place 2-3 drops on your wrists and the back of your neck before you study or read

- Emotional & spiritual grounding = use during prayer or mediation

- Soothing & uplifting = diffuse during a stressful season, or even during your morning commute (find a USB or travel diffuser)

- Makes a great addition to your skin care routine

- Wear as a cologne or personal scent

Odd fact, tidbit, random info: Two of the gifts the magi offered baby Jesus were essential oils, Frankincense and Myrrh. We see Frankincense featured throughout the Old Testament, as it's part of both the anointing oil and the holy incense. The word *incense* became so anonymous with the Frankincense in the ancient world that many times when you see the word the author is referring to Frankincense.

NOTES

LAVENDER

Relaxing

Unwind with a nighttime bath

Comforts skin

Diffuse for a peaceful environment

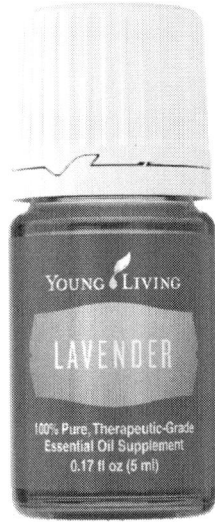

YOUNG LIVING

LAVENDER

100% Pure, Therapeutic-Grade
Essential Oil Supplement
0.17 fl oz (5 ml)

Single or blend: Single

Vitality: No, but Lavender Vitality is available at YoungLiving.com- many people use it for baking, as well as for internal support

Suggested uses:

- The relaxing aroma is great as part of a nighttime routine- diffuse before bed time or even when taking a nap

- Place 2-3 drops on the soles of your feet, inside your wrists, and the back of your neck before going to sleep

- May soothe fussy babies

- Place 2-3 drops on your skin when knicked, scratched, bruised, or blistered

Odd fact, tidbit, random info: Because of its many uses, Lavender is referred to as "The Swiss Army Knife of essential oils."

NOTES

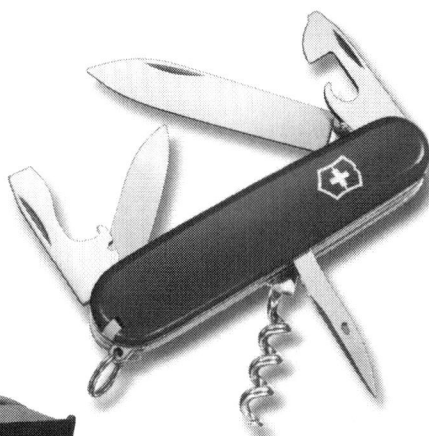

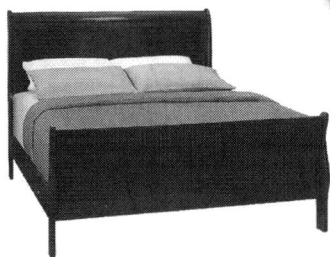

LEMON

Happy oil :-)

Great in food + drink

Goo-be-gone!

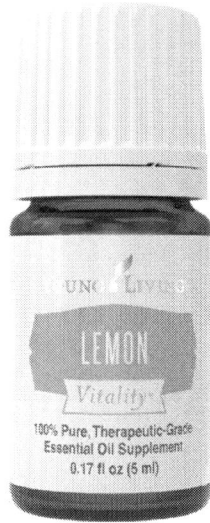

Single or blend: Single

Vitality: Yes

Suggested uses: Lemon is a powerful oil which is often overlooked because we're so familiar with *lemons*

- Comforts a tired or sore throat

- Place 2-3 drops in water or tea (hot or cold)

- Natural goo or stain remover

- Brightens your mood- so try diffusing it

- Place 1 drop on your toothpaste for brighter teeth

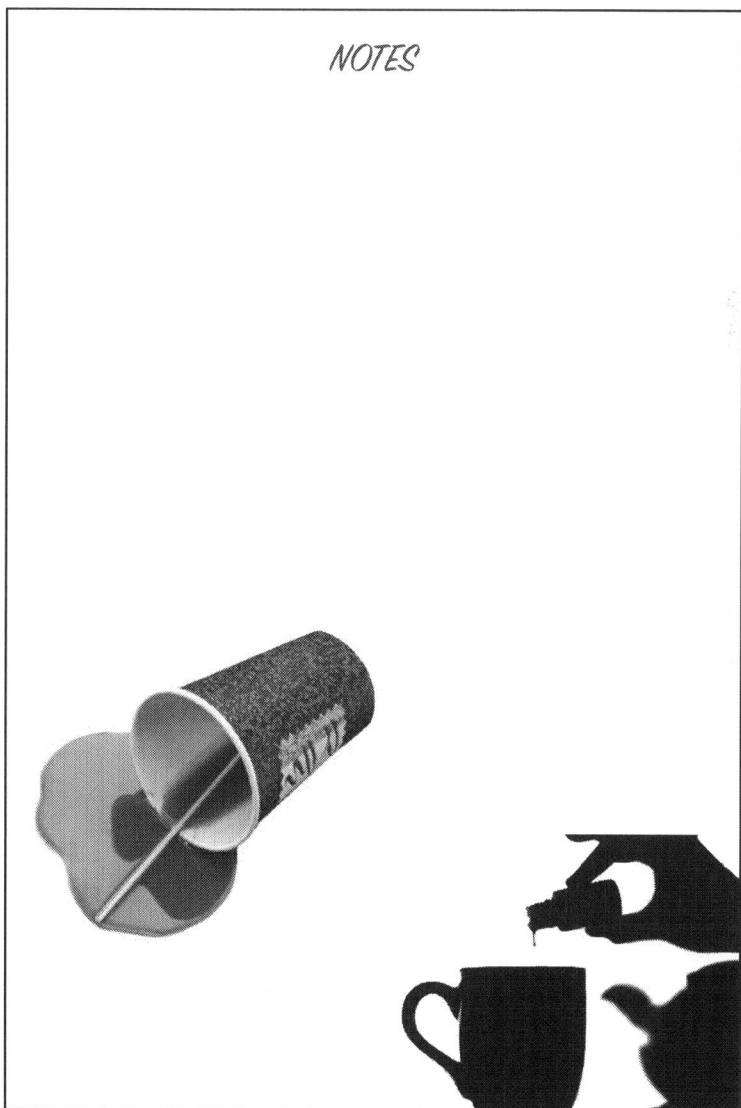

Odd fact, tidbit, random info: Lemon essential oil comes from the rind, not the juice.

NOTES

PANAWAY

Normal growing pains

Ligament + bone support

Same key ingredients as Agilease

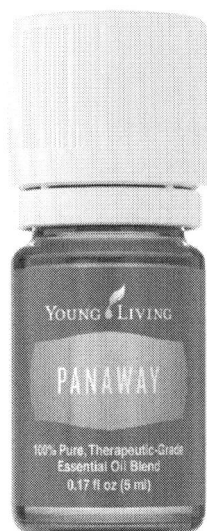

Single or blend: Blend

Vitality: No, and is not available as one

Suggested uses: Is a great oil for people of all ages- and all fitness levels

- Joints, ligaments, and muscles

- 2-3 drops with a carrier oil, massage into your skin, after a long run or an intense workout- use *before* you feel like you need it

- I know of lady that keeps this in her kitchen, in her car, and in her purse ("Perfect for aging bones and muscles," she says.)

- My oldest son swore by this one as he worked through that wretched season of growing pains (we made a roller bottle, using the age-recommended dilution)

Odd fact, tidbit, random info: Panaway is one of the few Young Living oils with a safety cap.

NOTES

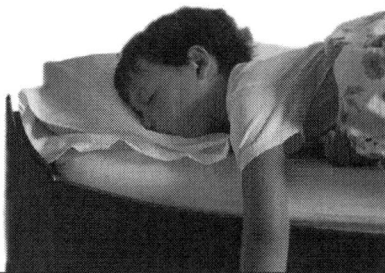

PEACE AND CALMING

Portable vacation

The name says it all

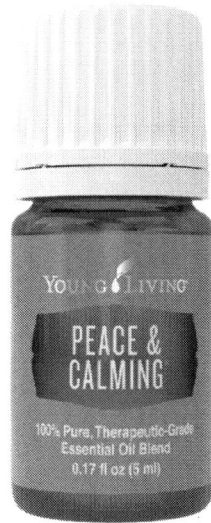

Single or blend: Blend

Vitality: No

Suggested uses:

- Carry this with you as an alternative to Stress Away (everyone is different, so some people prefer one oil and others prefer another)

- Diffuse in areas where your kids are when they need to "calm down" (we used to give our small boys a 5-minute "time out" near the diffuser, letting them breathe this oil)

- Make a rollerball for a sleepless child to keep nearby on nights they can't seem to get- or stay- asleep (also great as a prep for naps)

Odd fact, tidbit, random info: Peace & Calming was a staple in the Premium Starter Kit from 2013-2014. It was brought back by popular demand!

NOTES

PEPPERMINT

Motion queasiness?

Healthy bowel function

Afternoon slump

Great for exercise

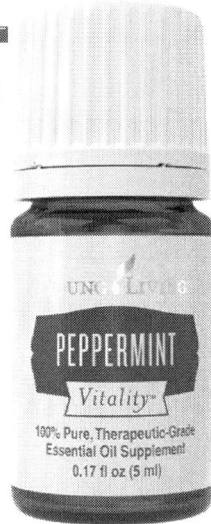

PEPPERMINT
Vitality™
100% Pure, Therapeutic-Grade
Essential Oil Supplement
0.17 fl oz (5 ml)

Single or blend: Single

Vitality: Yes

Suggested uses: You'll be shocked by the incredible versatility of this oil- it has as many varied uses as Lavender

- "Wake up" from an afternoon slump by diffusing this oil or by placing 2-3 drops in your water or tea (hot or cold)

- A great digestive support- use in the same ways as DiGize

- On hot days, place 1-2 drops behind each of your ears or on the back of your neck

- 2-3 drops on your forearms, at your pulse points, pre-workout, helps you get moving

- Inhale to open your breathing

- Use Peppermint to kick a bad coffee habit

Odd fact, tidbit, random info: Peppermint is green, and it smells nothing like the candy they give you at Mexican restaurants.

NOTES

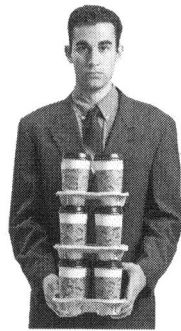

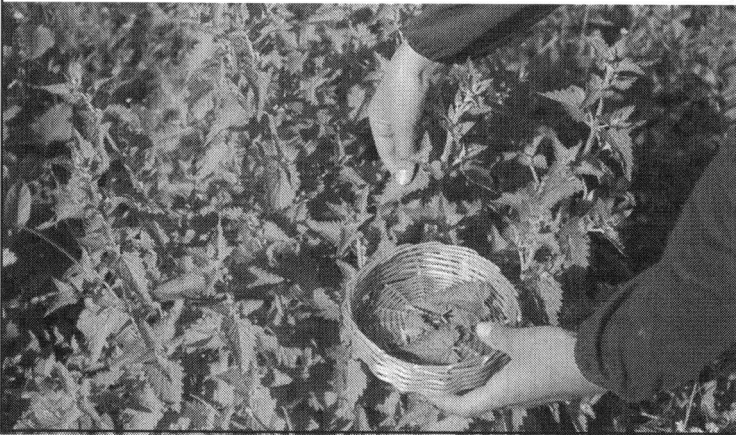

RAVEN

Rub on feet or chest before exercising to uplift and inspire

Diffuse to stimulate the senses

Cooling sensation on chest + throat

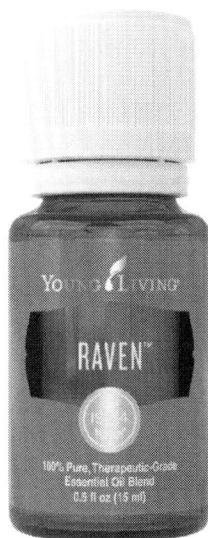

Single or blend: Blend, containing some of the best oils for breathing- Eucalyptus Radiata, Wintergreen, and Ravintsara

Vitality: No

Suggested uses:

- Incredible for respiratory needs

- Use proactively- not just when you feel like you need "help," but before you do (i.e., before you exercise)

- Provides a cooling sensation and soothing aroma when applied to your chest or throat

- Diffuse near you when you feel as if you need to open your lungs

Odd fact, tidbit, random info: This oil replaced R.C. in the PSK around Fall 2018. The two are virtually interchangeable.

NOTES

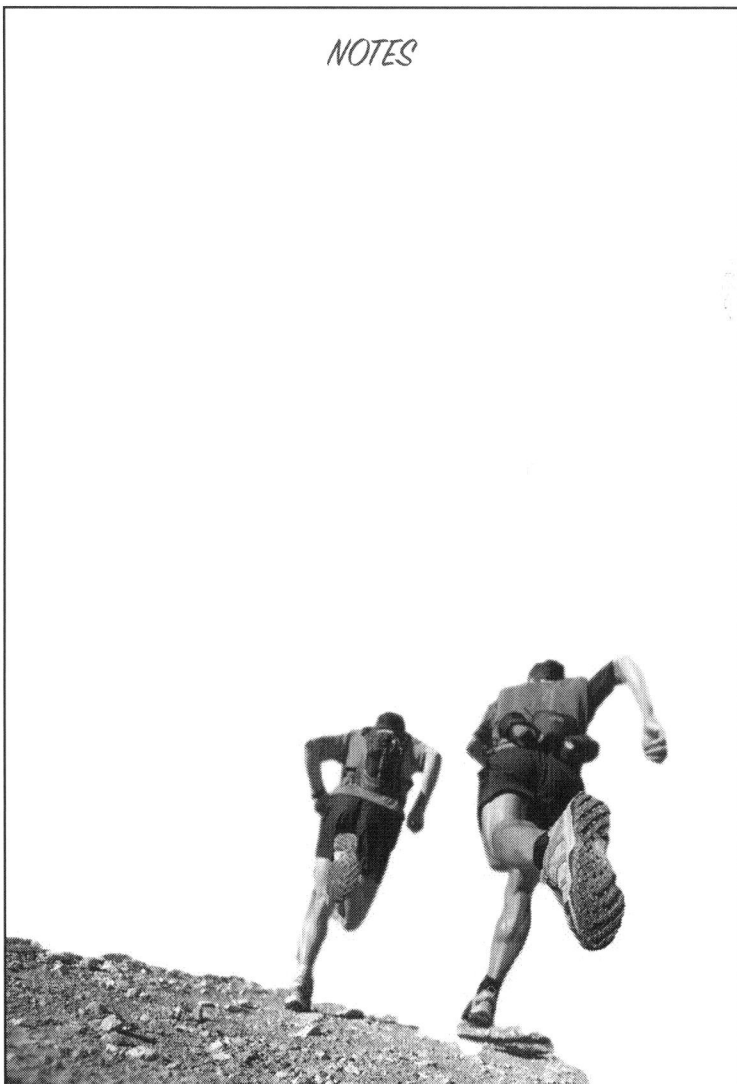

STRESS AWAY

Stress

Be

Gone

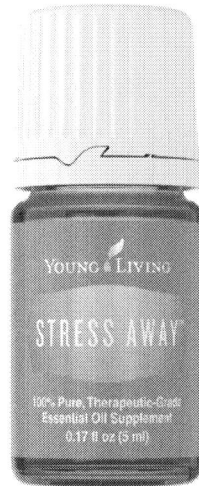

Single or blend: Blend

Vitality: No

Suggested uses: The name says it all

- Diffuse it everywhere you go- in your house, in your car, at your office, and even on a diffuser necklace or bracelet

- Carry this with you during times you need the emotional boost

- 2-3 drops on the inside of your wrists or on the back of your neck

- Place 2-3 drops in your palms, cup your hands, and breathe deeply for a micro-vacation from reality- or just inhale straight from the bottle

- Try Peace & Calming as an alternative. Some people respond better to one, others respond better to the other.

Odd fact, tidbit, random info: Contains Vanilla, which is known for enhancing relaxation.

NOTES

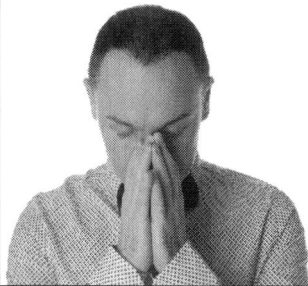

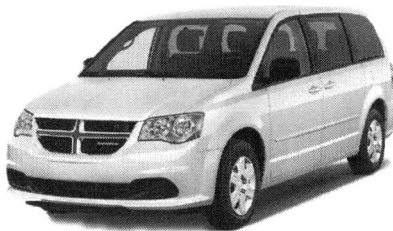

THIEVES

Heavy-hitter immune support

So powerful =
entire product line

Diffuse for added support

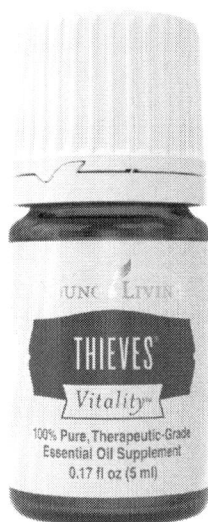

THIEVES
Vitality
100% Pure, Therapeutic-Grade
Essential Oil Supplement
0.17 fl oz (5 ml)

Single or blend: Blend, containing Cinnamon + Clove + Eucalyptus Radiata + Lemon+ Rosemary

Vitality: Yes

Suggested uses:

- Diffuse it in every room in your house- particularly during seasons when friends and coworkers are missing school & work with sickness

- Place 2-3 drops in a glass of water or (even better) in Ningxia Red and drink every day as part of your wellness routine

- Make your child a rollerball with the proper age-appropriate dilution so they have on-the-go support.

Odd fact, tidbit, random info: The story behind Thieves is fascinating. Learn more about it at OilyApp.com/AllThingsThieves.com.

As well, Young Living created an entire Thieves line based around this oil blend. For your second Young Living order (after the PSK) I highly recommend the Thieves ER kit. It's the best way to take a deep dive into the world of this immune support powerhouse!

NOTES

VALOR

Grounding when facing hard things

Valor = courage & bravery

Perfect when you've got to "step up" and get it done!

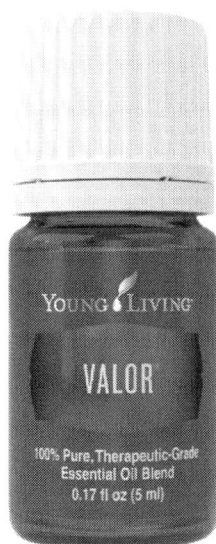

Single or blend: Blend

Vitality: No

Suggested uses:

- Diffuse when facing a hard day

- 2-3 drops on your neck or wrists, wear as a cologne or personal scent on days you need it

- Perfect for making a rollerball for children who play sports, have a tough time meeting new people, or walking into strange situations

- Massage on your back- is great for your skeleton

- Rub on the bottoms of your feet before going to sleep in order to give your partner a restful night of sleep :-)

Odd fact, tidbit, random info: Roman soldiers are said to have placed a similar blend of oils on the soles of their feet before marching into battle.

Notably, this is one of Young Living's most popular oils but was out of stock for years due to sourcing issues and the company's commitment to using only the highest quality ingredients.

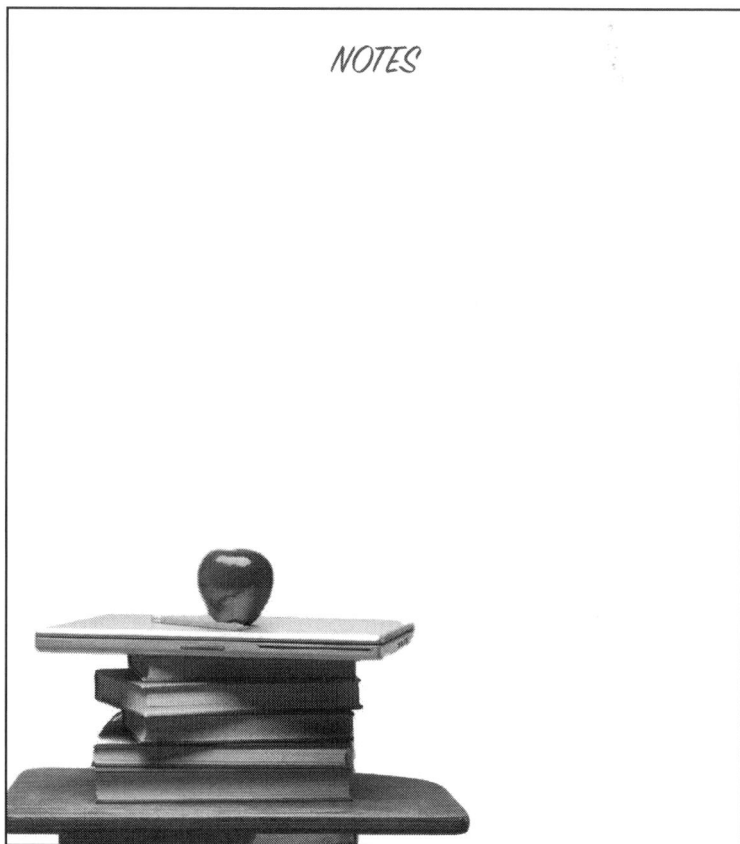

NOTES

12 OILS OF THE PREMIUM STARTER KIT

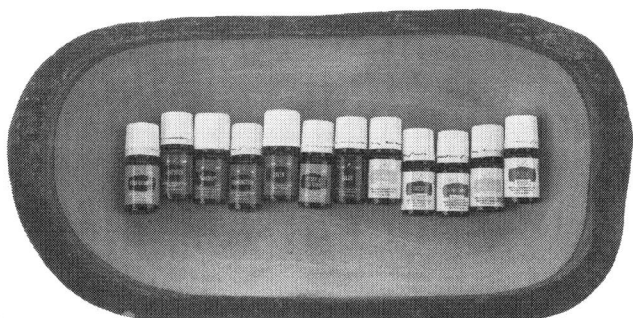

We just walked through the 12 oils of the Premium Starter Kit. Each essential oils PSK includes the oils and your choice of diffuser.

In addition, the kit contains two more products.

AND MORE

First, the PSK includes a concentrated package of Thieves Household Cleaner.

People interested in health routinely address issues with diet, supplementation, and essential oils- especially people like you who are more inclined to natural health solutions. However, we often neglect removing toxins from their environment.

It's easy to look at pics of the smog cloud that hovers over Los Angeles and think, "Yeah, that's a problem. Those people probably can't breathe too well. There's a lot of pollution there."

Or, we drive past the smoke stacks at a power plant or the industrial area of town and observe the same thing: "Too much junk in this environment to be healthy."

Intuitively we realize there are two major facets to our health:

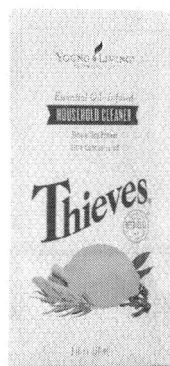

- Internal = what you place in your body (food, etc.)

- External = environment (what gets on you, where you live)

It's easy to complain about the environment "out there," something which we can't fix in the immediate. It requires a long-term solution, things which should begin now for sure, but something that will take time to achieve. At the same time, though, we radically under-estimate what we can achieve immediate in our own home.

Thieves Household Cleaner is one of the best ways to take charge of the environment you can control. And, it's far more economical that chemically-laden cleaners. The small packet in your PSK is concentrated, containing enough Thieves to make a full bottle.

.69¢ PER BOTTLE

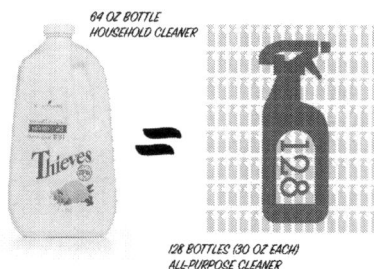

64 OZ BOTTLE
HOUSEHOLD CLEANER

128 BOTTLES (30 OZ EACH)
ALL-PURPOSE CLEANER

Second, the PSK includes 2 servings of Ningxia Red.

Ningxia is one of our "go-to" every single day choices for optimal health + wellness. I drink it by the shot, I mix it in shakes, I make home-made healthy Frappuccinos with it… you get the idea.

Here's why: whenever you use your muscles (whether you're working out or just living life) your cells go through a process called oxidization. That's a confusing word, but think of it like this: *oxidation is to your cells what rust is to muscles.*

(Some sources simply refer to aging as the compounded effect of oxidation + oxidation + oxidation.)

You need to get the rust off and get those things shiny and new again, right?

The end result = Feel stronger + look better with Ningxia Red.

All of this is included in the PSK. No worries if you're overwhelmed. In fact, after reading all of this you might be thinking, "I get it. I know how people get Sealed Kit Syndrome now. I know why that stuff stays in the box."

Ningxia Red comes in large bottles and in 2 ounce serving size packets.

Relax. In the next chapter, we've got you covered. We'll give you a sure-fire, time-tested way to make sure you break open that box and learn how to leverage the incredible goodness inside it.

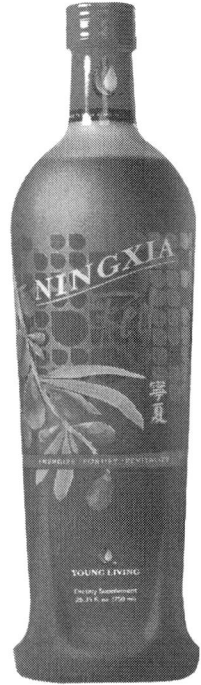

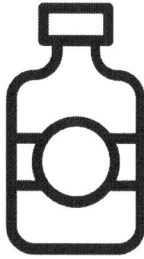

5 THINK INSIDE THE BOX

MAIN IDEA= THE BEST WAY TO START USING YOUR OILS IS TO... WELL... START USING YOUR OILS. WE CREATED THE 21 DAY CHALLENGE TO EMPOWER YOU TO MOVE FROM AN ESSENTIAL OIL NEWBIE TO A NATURAL HEALTH JUGGERNAUT IN JUST 3 WEEKS.

Thinking back about JB's infamous stashed away kit, I remembered how many times I'd taught health + healing workshops in church settings and bumped into the same thing. Inevitably, at the end of the 6-7 hour workshop (sometimes spanning a night and a morning), 1-2 people would always approach me with a similar scenario.

"I think I have one of these kits at home," someone would say," but I'm not sure."

Then, another- "I bought one- maybe- a few years ago at a party someone had in their house. I meant to use it. It sounded great. But I never got around to opening it up."

I heard stories about kits being stowed in linen closets, set atop refrigerators, and even placed with laundry detergents and cleaning supplies. It seems like a lot of people get these things and then forget what all they can do.

When I'm teaching a group class, I always have people who want to become new members complete a small form like the one included in the back of this book. They write their name, email address, and the other relevant info they need in order to become a new member, so that a few people I have running the computers can help them create their accounts and then return those forms to them. This makes the enrollment process move more rapidly and it insures the new member has the website and their login credentials written down for safe-keeping. (I can't tell you how many people we had to help call YL corporate to retrieve or reset their login before we started doing this!).

One day a sweet lady in her mid-fifties completed the form. It was a large class in which a lot of people decided to enroll as new members. She held that form and waited in line for about 30 minutes before she got to the front of the line.

After entering all of her personal info, meticulously typing every single bit of data, someone called for me.

"Hey, it seems like she's already a member. Young Living is asking her to login using her password."

"That doesn't make sense," I said. Then, after a few seconds, I decided to simply take it at face-value. She might actually already be a member I decided. I asked her, "Do you have one of these kits at home?"

"No."

"Are you sure?"

"I don't think I do?"

I waited.

Then, she spoke, as if she was processing it aloud. "You know, I've got a diffuser in the back bedroom that has that YL logo on it with the leaf, but I don't have those oils. Seems like we used to have a little box of 7 or 8 of them, but we never opened them. I haven't seen them for years."

We called customer service. Turns out, she was in the system. She purchased some oils a few years ago. And, though her account was no longer active, YL had a record that she'd bought from them before.

She bought some oils, but she never used them. Another example of Sealed Kit Syndrome. Like JB, she left her oils in the saran wrap. Unlike JB, though, she couldn't find hers.

THE OILYAPP 21 DAY CHALLENGE

"An ounce of prevention is worth a pound of cure."

I think Ben Franklin said it. He's the guy credited with it, anyway.

Here's what he means. If you can keep something from becoming an issue, that's better- and far more valuable- than dealing with the issue itself.

Why pay a full pound to fix something when you could have just invested an ounce in order to not ever mess with it in the first place?

That mantra is a great way to look at your health journey AND it's the way we need to look at your kit. Let's focus on health, not sickness- and focus on prevention instead of curing. And, as far as that box goes, I'll do some prevention that keeps you from getting "Sealed Kit Syndrome."

We call it the OilyApp 21 Day Challenge and the goal is simple: **move from Sealed Kit Syndrome to Oil-Slinging Syndrome in just three weeks.**

Here's how it works:

- Every day, for 21 days straight, we'll give you 3 super-quick, pleasantly practical things you can do to get familiar with your oils and your Young Living membership.

- Invest 10 minutes a day for the next 21 days to avoid Sealed Kit Syndrome. Check the boxes as you complete each task. [35]

- We'll even send you a certificate at the conclusion of the 3 week period, giving you the ability to showcase your achievement by sharing it on social media!

Don't have a smartphone or Internet access?

No worries. Keep reading. The 21 Day Challenge is included in the remainder of this chapter!

---

[35] You're free to complete this in any order. In fact, you might want to, depending on what health and personal concerns you wish to address. If you decide to work ahead, check everything off. Just make sure you complete all 60-plus tasks in 21 days.

THE **OilyApp** 21 DAY CHALLENGE

= THE BEST PREVENTION FOR SEALED KIT SYNDROME

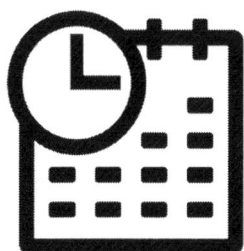

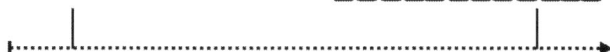

21 DAYS STRAIGHT + **3 THINGS / DAY**

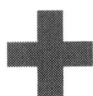

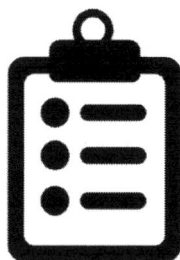

IN JUST 3 WEEKS!

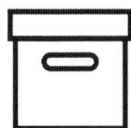

Sealed Kit Syndrome!

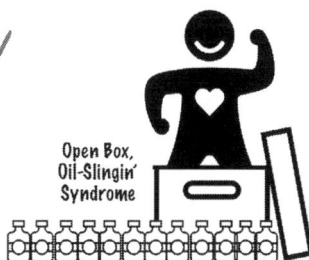

Open Box, Oil-Slingin' Syndrome

OH, NO!   **BOOYAH!**

Day 1: Open Your Box, Use Your Diffuser

Let's go ahead and insure we don't suffer from saran-wrapped kit syndrome by doing these few tasks.

- [ ] Find a quiet space (or at least an "empty space" like your kitchen table) and **open your PSK box**. Remove all of the contents and look through each of them. You'll find:

  - 12 essential oils

  - 2 servings of NingXia Red

  - A sample sachet of Thieves Household Cleaner

  - Roller bottle

  - Sample bottles & sample cards

  - Brochures from Young Living about the farms, the Seed to Seal process, and more

  Pro tip for using the sample bottles: At some point your kids are going to want your oils. Use the sample bottles to send them with a few drops of their favs to school, or even to keep in their bedroom.

  For his 11th birthday, one of my boys wanted his own PSK. I bought him a travel diffuser and loaded sample bottles for him. It was a much smaller investment, it was kid-sized and portable, and I could reload what he used the most. Plus, I didn't have to worry about him losing anything.

- [ ] **Open each oil, taking a few moments to smell all 12**. You're going to immediately love some of them. Others… not so much. Everyone is different. However, each oil in that kit has been specifically chosen for its therapeutic properties. Rest assured, they each have incredible uses. As you read this 21 Day Challenge, you'll learn more about each one.

☐ **Diffuse an oil.** When you find your favorite (fav for the moment), place 3-4 drops in your diffuser. Use tap water. The diffuser has a "fill line," so you don't overfill. Be sure it's plugged in, and turn it on. A few things to note:

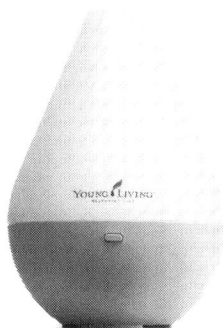

- Most diffusers have several light settings. Read the instructions or simply explore.

- Some have "full throttle" and intermittent settings (i.e., they'll diffuse for 30 seconds, then stop for 30, diffuse for 30, etc.). Again, read the manual or just tinker around.

- All of the diffusers have an automatic shut-off feature. This allows you to leave the house or go to sleep without worrying about burning up the motor. When the water runs out, they cut off.

☐ While you enjoy your diffuser, if you haven't already done so, go to www.OilyApp.com/ThinkInsideTheBox. **Watch the video** and register for the daily messages if you prefer to receive notifications on your smartphone.

Another pro tip: See if you can figure out how to set the display case up for your oils (the tray they are in lifts). This is a great way to set them on your counter, in your cabinet, or on a shelf. As well, once you raise that tray you'll see that there's a "secret compartment" in the bottom of the box which contains more literature and additional products.

Day 2: Empty the Box

By now you've had a chance to review the literature from our company, you've removed the saran-wrap from your box, and you've broken the seal on each of the bottles. Today, we'll keep working our way through the box.

☐ The first assignment for today is the same as the final task you did yesterday. **Open the oils again- each one- and *connect with the smell*.**

☐ **Remove the two Ningxia Red packets from your box and place them in your fridge.** We'll learn about Ningxia on Day 9.

☐ **Let's use the roller ball.** Find it in the "secret compartment" of your box. This will fit any YL oil bottle, so let's go ahead and use it. Place it on the Stress Away, then roll it across your forearms, your back, or your chest. Watch the video at OilyApp.com/Rollerball. (We'll learn more about this oil on Day 14.)

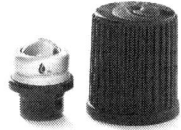

Pro tips for using the roller ball:

- Use the side of a key or a quarter to push your way between the top of the oil bottle and the bottle itself.

- Shimmy it off by holding the cap at an angle and rolling it around.

- To insure the roll ball is placed firmly on the bottle, screw the cap back on until you hear it click.

- Order empty bottles and roller balls from your VO or amazon.com, because you'll want to use the roller balls a lot- and changing the caps just isn't convenient!

- Roller balls are great for kids- zero chance of spillage!

Day 3: Citrus Fresh

Instead of your usual air fresheners, try diffusing Citrus Fresh today! It doesn't just cover up odors; it eliminates them!

☐ Take your diffuser to your bathroom- whichever one everyone in the house uses. Fill it with water, place 3-5 drops of Citrus Fresh in it, and leave it running all day. You'll need to refill it in a few hours.

Pro tip: You're going to want more diffusers. I have one in my living room, one in my bedroom, another in my restroom... I have one in just about every room.

You can find great diffusers in your Virtual Office, but you can also purchase them online or in other stores. Whereas the quality of your oils is critical, the type of diffuser you choose is largely up to you.

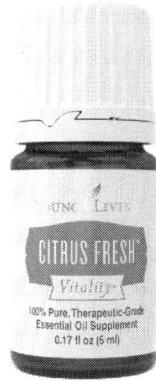

☐ **Place 2-3 drops of Citrus Fresh in your laundry today**, dropping it in the washing machine with the detergent you're currently using. Then, find some stinky shoes. Place 2-3 drops on a cotton ball and roll it inside each shoe.

☐ Citrus Fresh is one of the Vitality oils. **Place 1-2 drops in a glass of water and taste it.** I know people who put Citrus Fresh in their hot tea, others who place it in their Ningxia Red, and even others who place it in beer!

☐ Bonus step: **Review the three ways you can use essential oils from chapter 2-** touching (topically), smelling (inhaling), and tasting (ingesting)

Day 4: Digize

DiGize is the gold standard in digestive support. Notice, this is another Vitality oil.

☐ Before you eat dinner (or the largest meal you will eat today), **place 1-2 drops in a small glass of water and drink it**.

> Pro tip: Many people think about taking digestive supports only after they eat, but you can do this before you eat to help with bloating and healthy internal function.

☐ **After eating, place 2-3 drops of DiGize directly onto your stomach**.

Remember, even though the oils "travel" throughout our bodies, a general rule of thumb is to apply the oil as closely as you can to the area you want to reach. Do this same activity for any of your kids or others in your house who get a grumpy tummy.

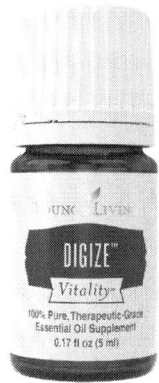

☐ DiGize has a unique smell. Remember, though, every oil in the PSK has been chosen specifically for its therapeutic benefits. **Flip to the notes space at the end of Day 7 and write your thoughts about DiGize.**

☐ Bonus step: DiGize is an oil I regularly use for my kids. **Review the dilution chart from chapter 2.** If you can, go ahead and make a diluted roller bottle for your kids.

> Pro tip: You can make your own capsules with DiGize and any of the Vitality oils. You can order them from your Virtual Office (VO) or from online stores.

Day 5: Frankincense

Frankincense is one of the most well-known essential oils. This is one of the three gifts the magi gave baby Jesus. You might not have thought of it as an essential oil in that story before, but that- and Myrrh- were both commonly used in the ancient world.

- ☐ **Frankincense is great for skin.** As part of your regular skin care routine, place 1-2 drops of the oil in your lotion today and see how it feels. If you don't use a lotion, just put a single drop in the palm of your hand. Then, use a finger to "dab it" on blemishes.

- ☐ **Diffuse 4-5 drops of Frankincense** as you reflect, read, or have a quiet time of meditation or prayer.

- ☐ **Place 1-2 drops on your wrists**. Inhale. Carry the bottle with you for the rest of the day, repeating this same activity whenever you need to refocus.

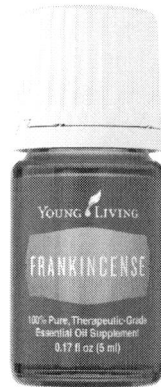

Pro tip: Frankincense also comes in a Vitality oil, meaning it has internal uses, as well!

Day 6: Lavender

Lavender is one of the most well-known essential oils. In fact, most of the pictures you see online related to oils are from lavender fields.

☐ **Carry your bottle of Lavender with you today**. Place a drop on your wrists and inhale whenever you need a brief "pause" for the day.

☐ Lavender is relaxing and peaceful. **Tonight before you go to bed, do the following:**

- Place 4-5 drops in your diffuser, in your bedroom, about an hour before bedtime. This will fill the room with the aroma.

- Just before bed, rub 2 drops on the bottoms of your feet, on your wrists, and the back of your neck.

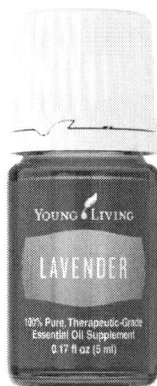

Pro tip: this is a great routine for Sunday afternoon naps, too.

☐ Lavender also comes as a Vitality oil. People place Lavender in lemonade, they bake cookies with lavender, they make cakes with lavender icing. The possibilities are endless. **Make a few notes of things you would like to try with Lavender:**

- _____

- _____

- _____

Day 7: Lemon

One of the most versatile oils is Lemon. It also happens to be one of the most over-looked. It's pressed from the rind- not made from the juice. Lemon soothes the occasional sore throat, energizes the body when added to your favorite drink, and even acts as a natural "goo-remover" for those tough messes, like gum and stickers.

☐ Lemon is one of the Vitality oils, meaning it's approved for internal consumption. **Try it for yourself!** Put 2 drops in a glass of water (only glass) and drink to enjoy improved mental clarity and energy.

☐ **Lemon is also a great goo-remover.** Place 2-3 drops on a damp cloth and then wipe away the mess. In addition to sticky globs like gum and grime, many people use Lemon to clean their knives, guns, and tools.

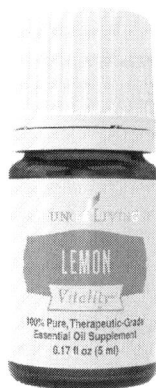

☐ Your PSK includes 12 oils- 5 are Vitality oils, 7 are "regular" oils. **Take at a look at your kit and list the 5 Vitality oils here**.[36]

1. _____

2. _____

3. _____

---

[36] You can find all of the Vitality oils at https://www.youngliving.com/en_US/products/c/essential-oil-products/dietary-essential-oils.

4. _____

5. _____

☐ **Bonus task:** Go to your Virtual Office at YoungLiving.com, use your user name and password to login, and search "Dietary Essential Oils," another name for Vitality. This will provide you with images of each of the current oils in the Vitality collection. Hint: you'll recognize Frankincense and Lavender are among this collection.

NOTES + JOTS + DOODLES

You've completed 7 days of the challenge! Place any of your notes + ideas here!

Day 8: Week 2, Monthly Promos & More

You've completed 7 days of tasks! You're 1 week into the 21-day challenge, 1/3 of the way through! Today, we want to review what you've learned, as well as look forward to what's planned for this week.

☐ **Monthly Promos** provide you with an incredible opportunity to receive free products every month. And, the more you purchase, the more free items you receive.

Here are two webpages for you to learn more about the promos.

- Go to OilyApp.com/MonthlyPromos (case-sensitive) to learn how monthly promos work, along with how you can combine them with Essential Rewards to get more bang for your buck!

- Young Living places their monthly promos on *this* page every month. It updates the first of every month: YoungLiving.com/en_US/opportunity/promotions/monthly-pv-promo.

Pro tip: bookmark the pages above and you'll never have to search to discover what the Monthly Promos are.

☐ The bottles in your PSK are all 5ml sizes. However, many of the oils are also sold in 15ml bottles. **Go to your virtual office at www.YoungLiving.com and login**, using the credentials you wrote down when you became a wholesale member. Take a look at the oils you've been using. **Place your 2 favorites in your shopping cart- as 15ml bottle**s. This will show you *how* to place an order. You can always remove them later- and you definitely don't want to order until we discuss Young Living's outstanding rewards program which gives you points back on every purchase you make.

☐ **Make note of your favorite uses of the 5 oils you've explored from your PSK.** And, be sure to continue with these uses even as you complete the challenges for the next 7 days.

- _____

- _____

- _____

- _____

- _____

☐ **Bonus assignment:** go on social media and tell your friends a story about your favorite product you used this week.

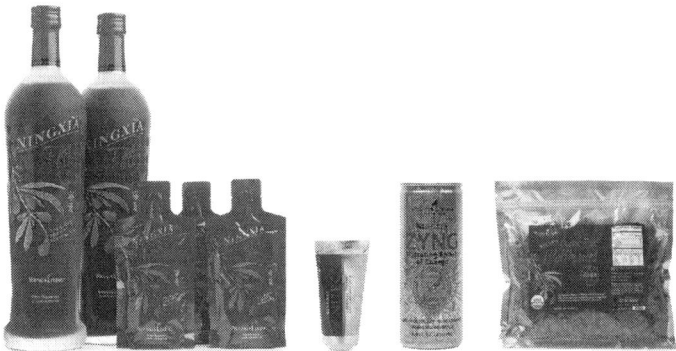

Day 9: Ningxia Red

Your PSK included 2 servings of Ningxia Red- YL's proprietary anti-oxidant drink. Today, let's learn a bit about Ningxia.

- ☐ **Take one of your Ningxia Packets out of the fridge and drink it!** You can drink it straight from the pouch or you can pour it into a cup or glass. 2 ounces is a full serving, so my kids regularly use "shot glasses" for consuming Ningxia.

- ☐ Go to OilyApp.com/Red (case-sensitive), **watch the short video**, and discover the benefits of YL's red drink.

- ☐ **Go to your VO and search "Ningxia."** I order the Ningxia ER kit every other month (and order the Thieves ER kit on alternating months). Write a few words on the following Ningxia products you find, noting how they might benefit you:

NINGXIA PRODUCTS

Ningxia Red (comes in bottles & 2 ounce "on the go" packets)

Nitro

Zyng

Wolf berries

Day 10: Panaway

Panaway is the only blend in your PSK which has a safety cap. Remember, safety caps are one of our "yellow lights" on our safety chart.

☐ Panaway is great for ligaments and joints for people of all ages.

- A 63-year old grandmother of 13 says she keeps one bottle in her purse, one on her bedside table, another on her kitchen counter, and one in the van. She applies it to joints and muscles and gives it to her friends!

- Youngsters like it, too. A 12-year old uses it to soothe normal growing pains, helping him sleep through the night comfortably.

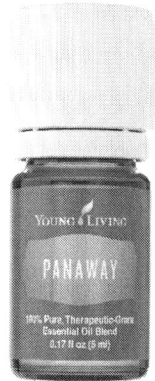

Apply 2-3 drops of Panaway to aching muscles, ligaments, or joints today. As well, if you see someone with a similar issue, offer some to them.

☐ Panaway can be used before you do manual work, walk, or exercise. In fact, most oils can be used *proactively-* to assist your body's normal healthy function. **Think of a way you can proactively use Panaway today- and then do so**. Note your results.

☐ **Review the information in this book about safety concerns** and essential oils (see chapter 2).

Day 11: Peace & Calming

Peace & Calming is another oil whose name says it all. This is a gem you'll find a lot of people carrying around with them as a "go to" on busy, hard-hitting days.

- ☐ **Use it for restful sleep.** Peace & Calming is another relaxing oil. In the same way you tried Lavender as a "sleep routine," do the same routine with Peace & Calming. Note which oil works for you, as everyone's body responds to them differently.

- ☐ **Carry this oil with you today**, using it in any of the following ways as you feel you need it:

  - Place 2-3 drops on your wrists and the back of your neck

  - Place 2 drops in your hand, cup them, and then inhale

  - Inhale the bottle directly

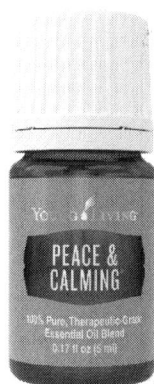

- ☐ **Use it for a "time out."** If you have small, busy kids (or any person of any age, for that matter) who could use a break, place 4-5 drops of Peace & Calming in the diffuser and set it near them. Place it on a table nearby, or even (as we did more than once!) place it on the floor and let them inhale it! Have them do so for 5 minutes, making note of the results.

  No one in the house? Do this for yourself!

Day 12: Peppermint

Peppermint is an oil with numerous uses. The first thing you'll notice about it, though, is that it doesn't smell at all like the "peppermint" candy they give you at the checkout counter in restaurants.

☐ Peppermint is another Vitality oil. **Today, put a drop in your water, hot chocolate, tea, or coffee.** You'll be blown away by its refreshing aroma and flavor.

Bonus: if you're baking brownies, place 4-5 drops in your batter.

☐ For a "wake up" in the middle of an afternoon or early evening slump, **place 3-4 drops of Peppermint in your diffuser.**

☐ Peppermint assists with healthy bowel function. Peppermint + DiGize pack a powerful one-two punch! Use it the same way you use DiGize.

☐ Peppermint also has a soothing, cooling effect. **On a hot day, place 1-2 drops behind your ears or on the back of your neck**.

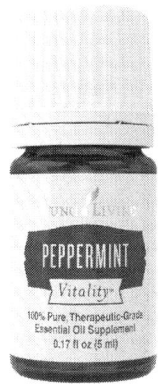

Pro tip: Peppermint is an athlete's favorite. Many use it before a workout to enhance their oxygen intake! I rub Peppermint on my forearms before working out or taking a long run.

Day 13: Raven

Breathing is a natural part of life. Raven can be such a blessing to support respiration. Open it, take a strong breathe of it, and experience the rejuvenating effects of Raven.

- ☐ **Try Raven before you exercise or take a walk**. Raven supports optimal respiratory function when applied to the chest. I went running with a few friends. I found out one of my friends- who seemed to run stronger than usual- applied Raven to his chest before we began.

- ☐ **Raven can also deliver a cooling sensation to your chest or throat.** Try 1-2 drops.

- ☐ **Diffuse Raven when you need to focus.** A high school teacher says, "I have been learning to use all sorts of combinations in my diffuser for my classroom. I took my diffuser home at one point and my high school students begged me to bring it back. They will even stand over it and try to breathe more of it in. They really love Raven."

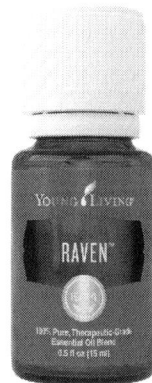

Pro tip: if you like Raven, try RC. At the end of 2018 Raven replaced RC in the PSK for supply chain reasons. RC is still available and is an incredible friend to your respiratory system.

NOTES + JOTS + DOODLES

You've completed 13 days of the challenge! Place any of your notes + ideas here!

Day 14: Stress Away

We often refer to Stress Away as a "vacation in a bottle".

☐ **Place 3-4 drops of Stress Away in your diffuser and set it near you, where you can enjoy the aroma**. Make note of how you feel after just a few minutes.

☐ If you're starting your day, place the bottle of Stress Away in your pocket or purse and **carry with it you for the day.** If you're ending your day, carry it tomorrow. Be sure to set aside a few a times when you can use it (i.e., set mental reminders, such as when you take your coffee break, when you step on the elevator, lunch break, etc.). Great usage tips include:

- Placing a few drops on your wrists and rubbing them together

- Placing a few drops on your hands, cupping them, and then inhaling

- Inhaling straight from the open bottle

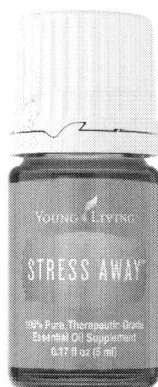

Pro tip: if you have a car diffuser, Stress Away makes a great commuting companion.

☐ **Find someone at home or work you can share your Stress Away with.** Just let them know what you did and how it made you feel, letting them know that they looked like they could use it!

Day 15: Week 3, Review + Reference Tools

Congratulations on completing 2 full weeks of the 3 week challenge. Today, we're going to review what you've learned, as well as tell you about an amazing organization YL has created.

☐ **Go to OilyApp.com/OilyApp.** Our app turns your smartphone into an essential oil pocket reference guide. Take a look and see if it would be helpful for you on your journey. It's a one-time fee purchase, and includes some of our tips on how to use the oils.

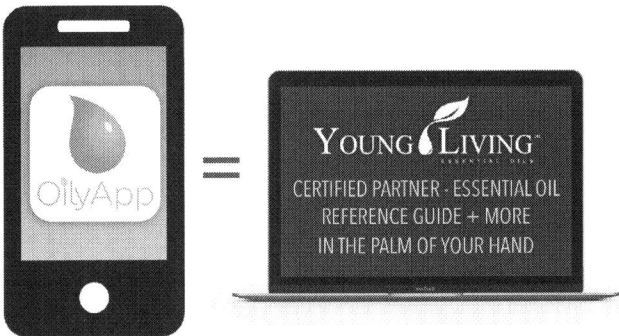

☐ You've used 10 of the 12 oils so far. We only have Thieves and Valor to go. **Take a few moments to make notes about your "go to" oils- and your favorite ways to apply the oils you've used.**

- _____

- _____

- _____
- _____
- _____
- _____
- _____
- _____
- _____

☐ **The founder of Young Living, Gary Young, launched a charitable foundation years ago.** Young Living covers all of the operational expenses, allowing 100% of the donations to go to direct, hands-on work the foundation does around the world.

- Learn more at YoungLivingFoundation.org

- You can also download several OilyApp+ podcast episodes where we discuss the foundation with foundation ambassadors, as well as the Executive Director. Go to the OilyApp.com/blog webpage and look for episodes 57, 60, & 65. Search the OilyApp+ podcast on Apple Podcasts or wherever you listen to podcasts.

☐ **Bonus assignment. Share what you're learning!** Go on social media and tell your friends one thing you learned about Young Living or a story about one product you used this week.

Day 16: Thieves (Oil Blend)

Thieves is the ultimate immune support! And, it's one of Young Living's most popular oils.

☐ Thieves comes in both the Vitality (white label) and "regular" (colored label) versions. The Thieves in your PSK is one of the 5 Vitality oils (the others are Citrus Fresh, DiGize, Lemon, & Peppermint). **Try Thieves in one of the following ways today:**

- 1- 2 drops in Ningxia Red

- 1-2 drops in hot tea or coffee

- 1-2 drops in a small glass (3-4 ounces) of water

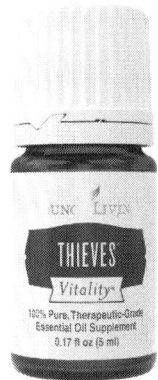

☐ **Diffuse Thieves** this evening as everyone unwinds from their day.

☐ **Watch the video at OilyApp.com/AllThingsThieves** (URL is case-sensitive). This will help you understand more about where Thieves originated, as well as how to use the Thieves blend.

Pro tip: This book is #5 in our series of "books you'll actually read." The previous book is All Things Thieves. You can find it at OilyApp.com/books or you can download it free in the OilyApp+ membership portal. Go to OilyApp.com/plus for more info.

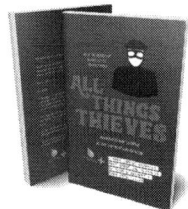

Day 17: Thieves Household Cleaner

Thieves essential oil is so powerful that Young Living developed an entire line of household and personal products based on this must have oil. The Thieves Household Cleaner is concentrated.

Your PSK includes a small sachet with enough cleaner to make a full bottle. Today, do the following:

☐ **Watch the video** at OilyApp.com/ ThievesCleaner to learn more about the importance of using all natural cleaning products in your home.

☐ Find an empty spray bottle (or make a trip to Walmart, the Dollar Tree, or another nearby store and purchase one), so that you can **mix your Thieves Household Cleaner today.**

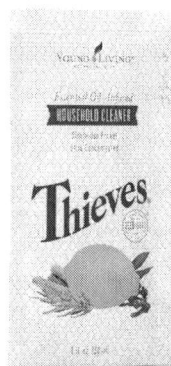

Pro tip: I use Thieves Household Cleaner to clean everything in my house-from the doors to the floors. And, I use it to clean my car. We have a dilution chart on the OilyApp.com/ThievesCleaner webpage, as well as a cost comparison. You'll find this is an economic alternative with radical versatility.

☐ **Login to your Virtual Office and search "Thieves."** You'll find yourself surprised at how many Thieves products YL has created. While you're there, look for the Thieves Essential Rewards Kit. This is a product I order every other month, in order to keep inventory of healthy versions of items I use almost every day: household cleaner, toothpaste, laundry soap, dish soap, etc.

Day 18: Valor

Rumor has it that Roman soldiers used a blend similar to Valor before marching into battle. This is a perfect metaphor, because courage- or valor- only exists in the context of facing hard things.

☐ **Identity someone in your family who could use an extra dose of courage today.** Perhaps a child is facing a test, an appointment, or a sporting event and could use a boost. Or maybe you're facing a tough conversation, a task at work, or something else you've been putting off. Open your bottle of Valor and have the person- or you- inhale it deeply. Place 2-3 drops on the wrists, as well as a drop on the back of the neck. Valor is also great to diffuse. If you have time, diffuse Valor at the start of your day- or even before whatever you're facing.

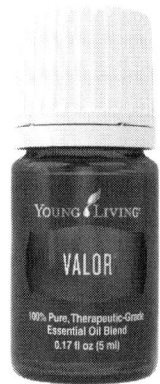

☐ **Valor is great to massage onto your back and spine.** Take a few drops and do so.

☐ Valor also comes as a Roll-On oil. Go to your Virtual Office at YoungLiving.com, use your user name and password to login, and **search "Roll-Ons."** This will show you the current collection of Roll-On oils.[37]

---

[37] Or search at https://www.youngliving.com/en_US/products/c/essential-oil-products/roll-ons.

Day 19: Explore To Learn More

Today we're going to do some online exploration. I'll point you to three resources where you can discover even more about the wonderful world of essential oils and oil-infused products.

- ☐ Login to your VO. **Look for "YL University."** This is an incredible- and free- resource that many people overlook!

- ☐ One of the greatest attributes of YL is the commitment to product integrity. This is all encapsulated in the Seed to Seal process. We discussed that in our book, but there are videos you can find at SeedToSeal.com. **Take a few minutes to explore the Seed to Seal site.**

- ☐ There are a *ton* of niche interests in Young Living. You'll find that people focus on everything from pets to emotions to athletics to personal care and more. Here are a few items that may be of interest to you.

  Choose something that interests you below and watch the video on that page (URLs below are all case-sensitive).

  - Athletes = OilyApp.com/pskathletes

  - Emotions and emotional health using oils = OilyApp.com/AFTZoomReplay

  - Oils of the Bible = OilyApp.com/BibleOils

  - Pets = OilyApp.com/Pets

Day 20: Essential Rewards (ER)

Essential Rewards (ER) is Young Living's frequent buyer program. We've referred to it a few times over the past 19 days.

Here's how it works: You select the products you want, you choose your ship date, and you're not locked into buying stuff you don't want or things you won't ever use. Plus, the program pays you back!

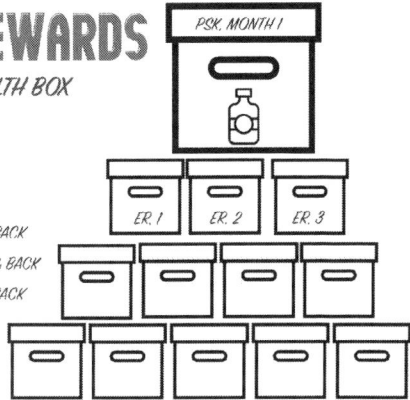

ESSENTIAL REWARDS
= OPTIONAL MONTHLY HEALTH BOX
* NOT AUTOMATIC
* FREQUENT BUYER
* POINTS BACK! MONTHS 1-3 = 10% BACK
             MONTHS 4-24 = 20% BACK
             25+ MONTHS = 25% BACK
* FREE GIFTS!
* DISCOUNTED SHIPPING

Here are today's assignments:

☐ Login to your VO, find the Essential Rewards tab, and **enroll as a member of this free program**- if you haven't already done so. Place your 3 favorite oils in the shopping cart, as well as one more product you'd like to try.

☐ **Young Living has bundled a few Essential Rewards kits.**
The two I purchase most frequently are the Thieves ER kit and the Ningxia Red ER kit. I alternate months, purchasing one 60 days. While you're in your VO take a look at each of these kits and think about how they might serve you and your family.

☐ **We wrote a 15 page eBook you can download absolutely free**. It tells you how to leverage the Monthly Promos (Day 8) and Essential Rewards to:

- Receive the best price possible on all of the products

- Receive free products each month that Young Living wants you to try

- Earn points towards free products you choose

- Earn even more points towards more free items the longer you're a member of this optional program

- Receive the best price on shipping

- Choose healthier alternatives for your family without spending more (in fact, you may spend less!)

We've placed the info at OilyApp.com/ER for you.

Day 21: Ditch & Switch

Young Living is more than "just essential oils." The company has over 500 healthy products, all designed to empower you to walk in health and wholeness.

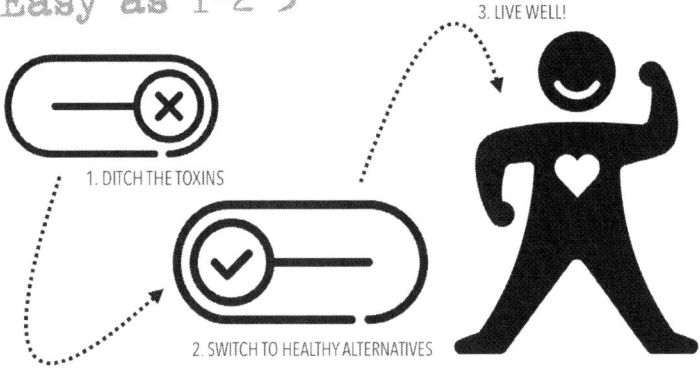

Easy as 1-2-3

1. DITCH THE TOXINS

2. SWITCH TO HEALTHY ALTERNATIVES

3. LIVE WELL!

☐ The best way to pursue a healthier lifestyle is to leverage ER to:

- Eliminate unhealthy products you currently use

- Replace them with healthy alternatives

We created a "Ditch & Switch" worksheet to help you make the switch. The PDF allows you to look at the products you currently buy and then discover Young Living's alternative. Get the document- free of charge- at OilyApp.com/ditchNswitch.

☐ **Using the worksheet, identify 3 products you can swap now**. With everything from makeup to supplements, from household products to cooking collections, Young Living has you covered. Place those products in your ER cart.

☐ **Share the link to the Ditch & Switch on social media worksheet, letting friends know one thing you learned!**

NOTES + JOTS + DOODLES

You've completed ALL 21 days of the challenge! Place any of your notes + ideas here!

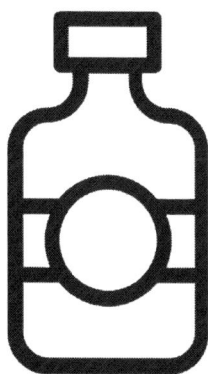

APPENDIX

YOUR NEXT BEST STEP

Thanks for joining us on that journey through *Essential Oils 101*.

At this point, you find yourself in one of two groups.

- **Group 1 = you're already a Young Living member.** If so, it's time to make sure you've broken through Sealed Kit Syndrome and that you're leveraging the full benefits of your membership through Essential Rewards. If you haven't already done so, join the 21 Day Challenge as printed in the book- or register for daily updates at OilyApp.com/ThinkInsideTheBox.

- **Group 2 = you're not a member yet, but you're super-excited to get started!** The best place to begin is to order your Premium Starter Kit.

If someone invited you to a class or handed you this book, please refer to them for their member number. Ordering through YoungLiving.com with their member number will insure that you're on their team and can work in close relationship with them.

If you stumbled upon this material by "accident," PM / DM us @OilyApp from any social media platform or text 205-291-1391 and we'll help you get started!

COMMON TERMS

Here are four commonly used terms, particularly related to the PSK:

Single- A single is an oil that comes from one plant. Frankincense, Lavender, Lemon, and Peppermint are all singles.

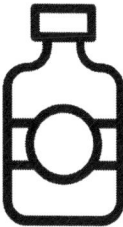

SINGLES

Essential Oils are the life source of the plant. You can use them in three ways- touch them, inhale them, or swallow them (Vitality labeled only).

Singles come from one plant.

Blend- Blends come from multiple plant sources. Some oils work well together. For convenience, Young Living produces many blends. Citrus Fresh, DiGize, Panaway, Peace & Calming, Raven, Stress Away, Thieves, and Valor are all blends that come with your PSK. You'll likely find yourself experimenting with your own blends. Every oil you have is either a single or a blend- but not both.

BLENDS

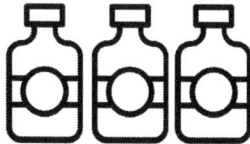

Some oils work incredibly well together. So, Young Living "blends" them before you receive them. It removes the guess work, while making it super simple to use them.

Blends come from multiple plants.

Vitality- Vitality is a trademarked term by Young Living. Vitality oils have been approved for human consumption by the FDA. Vitality oils may be singles or blends. They are easy to recognize, as they have white labels which closely resemble their non-Vitality counterparts.

VITALITY

Vitality oils are certified and approved by the FDA for human consumption.

Vitality Oils, a trademarked name by Young Living, have white labels w/ the same color trim as their non-Vitality counterparts.

Oil infused product- An oil infused product is an everyday item that contains essential oils in it, in order to enhance its health benefits.

Young Living carries 500+ different items in their inventory. You'll find everything from supplements to household products to dietary products (i.e., shakes, some foods), to personal care products and more.

OIL INFUSED PRODUCTS

Oils can be used to cook, to clean... for your pets... in soaps+ shampoos... in just about every room in your home.

Oil-infused products come in all shapes + sizes- for every facet of your healthy lifestyle.

HOW TO RUN YOUR OWN CLASS

We wrote Essential Oils 101 with a specific mindset.

First, we asked the following question: *What if we had a new member in our organization, but we could never speak to them, yet we wanted to be certain they had access to all of the information they would ever need in order to effectively launch their Young Living journey?*

Now, neither one of us are about to "not talk" to anyone- particularly someone who's part of our business organization. At the same time, though, putting that question on the table forced us to focus and define a few things. We needed to write down-

- Specific things we wanted to tell that person about essential oils

- Why Young Living was the best choice

- How to use those products (and avoid Sealed Kit Syndrome)

- How to order more while getting the best price and benefiting from the incredible rewards program Young Living offers

- How to navigate their Virtual Office for additional info

- Where to learn about the other products YL offers, and how to "Ditch & Switch" to them.

- How to best train them if we were unable to speak

Hopefully, we've covered all of that- and a bit more.

Second, we asked ourselves a follow-up question: *What if they wanted to train someone- could we create a way for them to do that, assuming we wouldn't be able to talk to either one of them?*

Again, it's purely hypothetical. We're both extremely accessible, but it got us thinking about how we could coach someone to lead others on the same journey.

That said, here's how we encourage you to move forward:

1. **Read and re-read this book and watch + rewatch the accompanying videos** for the May 2019 editor of OilyApp+ - login at OilyApp.com/login if you're a member or register at OilyApp.com/plus.

2. **Complete the 21 Day Challenge for yourself.** Even if you've been in essential oil world for years, you'll want to know what you're sending you friends to do. (Plus, we'd love your feedback, as well as things we can do to make it even better!)

3. **Order enough books to have on-hand for everyone you hope will attend your class.** You can find them on Amazon or at OilyApp.com/books.

4. **At the beginning of your class, pass the books to everyone- just as we described in the introduction**. Let them know that the books are yours and that they can pass them in when the class concludes- but that you're going to give a book to anyone who purchases their kit.

5. **During the class, don't read the book to them!** The purpose of step 1 is to become so familiar with the contents of this book that you don't need to read it. Rather, this book simply serves as an outline, your guide, something to point them to.

6. **Know where you're going to go during your class.** Have the pages in your copy of the book dog-eared, and be ready to skip around. Suggestion for a 45 minute class:

   - 5 minutes in chapter 1, defining what essential oils are

   - 5 minutes in chapter 2, discussing the 3 ways you can use them (touch, smell, taste)

   - 2 minutes talking about quality from chapter 3

   - 3 minutes defining the terms in chapter 1 (single, blend, Vitality, and oil infused products)

   - 25 minutes or less walking through the 12 oils in chapter 4

   - 5 minutes closing the sale

7. **Be sure to ask them to purchase a kit and invite them to join Essential Rewards during the close.** You'd be shocked at how many people teach an incredible class and skip this part!

8. **We've included an "order form" on the following pages.** Rather than have people sit at the computer and look for their credit card, try to create a login, and come up with a PIN and password while sitting at the computer to order, have them

complete the form first. The info will remain in this book (which will be theirs to keep), insuring they have a safe place to remember their login credentials!

9. Encourage them to join the 21 Day Challenge, too. They can use the book you've gifted them with their purchase or they can register- free of charge- online at OilyApp.com/ThinkInsideTheBox.

By the way, if you're interested in team building, access the "Work It!" compensation plan series at OilyApp.com/WorkIt (URL is case-sensitive). The series is free for OilyApp+ members.

ORDERING INFO

Instructions: complete the following info and then go to YoungLiving.com to become a member. This will help you navigate the site more easily and it will provide you with a written record of your login credentials.

NAME

STREET

CITY

STATE   ZIP

PHONE

EMAIL

USERNAME

PASSWORD 8-12 characters (A-Z, a-z & 0-9)   PIN (4 digit #)

CREDIT CARD #

CVV # found on the back of the card   EXPIRATION

ENROLLER NAME (the person who invited you)   ENROLLER # (discount code!)

CUSTOMIZE YOUR PREMIUM STARTER KIT

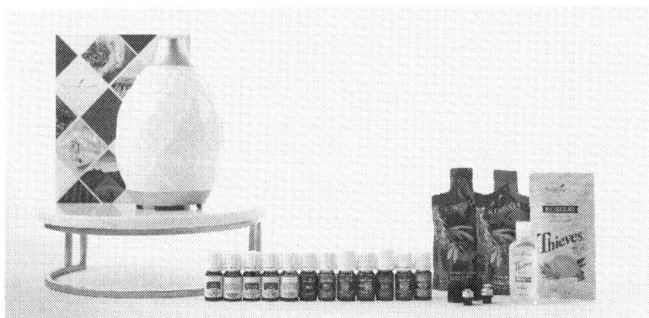

PREMIUM STARTER KIT INCLUDES

* 12 oils (as pictured)
* Plus your choice of Desert Mist diffuser ($165) or (select below)

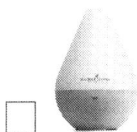

☐ **$165 PSK**
w/ Dew Drop diffuser

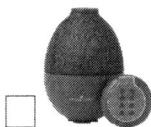

☐ **$210 PSK**
w/ Rainstone diffuser

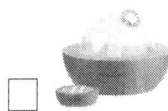

☐ **$265 PSK**
w/ Aria diffuser

SOME OF OUR FAVORITE MUST HAVES!

ESSENTIAL REWARDS KITS
Earn the benefits of ER right away!

☐ THIEVES ER KIT - $118.50

☐ NINGXIA RED ER KIT - $187

WEB LINKS

Throughout this book we provided you with several webpages where you can find more info and take a deep dive into the wonderful world of essential oils.

Links specific to this book

- For info about this book and ordering information, go to OilyApp.com/101

- To register for the free 21 Day Challenge and avoid Sealed Kit Syndrome, visit OilyApp.com/ThinkInsideTheBox

OilyApp resources

- App = OilyApp.com/OilyApp or search your app store

- Books = OilyApp.com/books (to buy in bulk or link to Amazon)

- OilyApp+ = ongoing education = OilyApp.com/plus

- Podcast = OilyApp.com/blog (links to providers here, or stream online) or search OilyApp+ in your favorite podcast provider

21 Day Challenge links (note: our URLs are all case-sensitive)

- Comp plan series = OilyApp.com/WorkIt

- Ditch & Switch worksheet = OilyApp.com/ditchNswitch

- Essential Rewards, 15 page eBook & video = OilyApp.com/ER

- Monthly Promos, explanation = OilyApp.com/MonthlyPromos

- Ningxia Red = OilyApp.com/Red

- Rollerball tops = OilyApp.com/Rollerball

- Special interest, Bible Oils = OilyApp.com/BibleOils

- Special interest, emotional health = OilyApp.com/AFTZoomReplay

- Special interest, pets = OilyApp.com/Pets

- Special interest, sports = OilyApp.com/pskathletes

- Thieves, all products = OilyApp.com/AllThingsThieves

- Thieves Household Cleaner = OilyApp.com/ThievesCleaner

Young Living webpages to bookmark

- Main page = YoungLiving.com

- Monthly Promos (updates every month) = YoungLiving.com/en_US/opportunity/promotions/monthly-pv-promo

- Seed to Seal = SeedToSeal.com

- Young Living Foundation = YoungLivingFoundation.org

OilyApp plus

Want to watch the videos that go with this book? And other videos?

OilyApp+ was created for you!

OilyApp+ is a web-based monthly membership / subscription service which provides you with each of the following:

- A monthly class- including a downloadable script AND the videos for the material in this book

- Graphics to match the class!

- 60 second videos to review each of the products mentioned in the class

- Access to Diamond+ leaders and biz-building tips

- Bonus classes taught by Dr. Jim Bob

And, it's incredibly affordable. In fact, as we often tell people, it's super-smart, pleasantly practical, and costs less than a latte!

Join the movement at www.OilyApp.com!

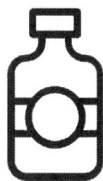

Unless you've been hiding like a hermit for the past few years, you've probably heard of essential oils. You've seen them in stores, you've watched parents use them on their kids, and you've seen ladies carrying huge clear bags with them prominently displayed. You might have even attended a "house party" and been asked to "sign up."

Geez, you might have an unopened kit sitting atop your fridge or tucked away in the back bedroom. Maybe it even intimidates you!

But what are these oils? And do they really work?

In *Essential Oils 101*- our 6th book you'll actually read- we go back to the basics. We think the oils are extraordinary, out-of-this-world awesome. But, we make them super-simple and pleasantly practical between the these covers.

We'll answer all the questions you have, questions like-

- *What are they and do they really work?*

- *Is there really a difference between what I can get at the grocery store and what I buy online?*

- *Are they safe? And what can they do?*

As a bonus, we include our proprietary 21 Day Challenge. You can follow along in the book, or you can register online for daily updates delivered to your smartphone. We'll work with you to break the "Sealed Kit Syndrome" and make sure you know what, how, when, where, and why to use those oils!